THE MODERN FASTING DIET PLAN

The Beginners intermittent fasting guide to loss weight and Feel Better step-by-step.

By David Johnson

Book 1

Book 2

Chapter 1. Introduction

There are a huge number of books composed on the point presenting distinctive eating less junk food plans for weight reduction clarifying the absolute most well-known sustenance approaches and considerably more. A considerable lot of these weight control plans propose removing certain macros, for example, cutting carbs or fats. Some of them recommend people should cut their everyday calorie admission, some propose an increment in active work.

There is without question a ton of going on, yet there is eadditionally one key factor which is absent in these eating less junk food plans. That factor is fasting, which is an experimentally demonstrated technique for bringing numerous medical advantages, assisting with weight reduction and significantly more.

Numerous individuals accept that fasting is tied in with starving, yet this isn't the situation. When fasting is done appropriately, it is one of those astoundingly powerful methodologies which can create stunning outcomes paying little mind to which eating less junk food plans you embrace.

1.1 What is Intermittent Fasting?

Intermittent fasting is a vague term for cycling between times of fasting and eating. There are a few kinds of intermittent fasting, yet they all offer one significant shared trait: Instead of zeroing in principally on what you eat, you focus harder on when you eat (albeit that doesn't mean the nature of your eating regimen isn't likewise significant).

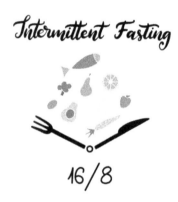

As indicated by Dr. Imprint Mattson, an analyst on intermittent fasting and teacher of neuroscience at Johns Hopkins University, the human body is intended to abandon nourishment for a few hours to a few days, however after the Industrial Revolution, food became available constantly. Subsequently, the human eating regimen changed altogether, and science hasn't got up to speed yet. Individuals are eating more food all the more regularly, and these additional calories (combined with stationary ways of life) have prompted ongoing medical problems like stoutness, type 2 diabetes, and coronary illness, which is the main source of death for ladies in the United States. At the point when you go for set timeframes without food, it permits your body to appropriately zero in on assimilation and exhaust your energy or glucose stores so your digestion is compelled to begin consuming your own muscle to fat ratio. Matt-child characterizes this cycle as "metabolic.

Intermittent fasting is a genuinely remedial methodology which can bring staggering outcomes in regards to weight reduction progress and by and large, both physical and emotional well-being in individuals who choose to accept it. Those people who are worn out on continually tallying their everyday calorie consumption, who are burnt out on fixating on the food sources they burn-through and who are basically worn out on disposing of their number one food sources from their eating routine, ought to clearly think about accepting the intermittent fasting way of life.

There are various advantages brought by an intermittent fasting way of life and one of them is that you don't need to surrender your number one food varieties helpful for arriving at your ideal weight and in compatibility of feeling incredible.

With intermittent fasting, people, truth be told, change their eating designs, they change when they eat, yet not what they eat. Consequently, there is no compelling reason to remove your number one food varieties, to stay away from delectable desserts and different food sources which are much of the time kept away from when following other well-known slimming down plans.

There is no more calorie tallying, no more fixating on your food sources and not any more battling with remaining progressing nicely. With intermittent fasting, you, truth be told, change your way of life adopting a straightforward steady strategy, you study eating fewer carbs propensities, their significance for your general wellbeing lastly, you figure out how to accept intermittent fasting for various medical advantages.

Regardless of your explanations behind being here, intermittent fasting is the best approach whether you need to normally get in shape, support your digestion, increment your energy or just feel incredible and sound each day.

To numerous individuals, intermittent fasting may seem like an exceptionally prohibitive methodology, as many accept that it is tied in with starving yourself, not eating routinely and other comparably false convictions. The book will break those false convictions. It will bring what you need to know on intermittent fasting, its medical advantages just as a basic, yet compelling bit by bit approach you can take helpful for benefiting from this slimming down way of life.

With the book, you will likewise find what the science is behind intermittent fasting backing up those various intermittent fasting benefits for your wellbeing. Furthermore, interestingly, you don't have to deny yourself of your best food sources for arriving at your wellbeing and counting calories objectives.

Intermittent fasting additionally furnishes stunning outcomes when joined with another mainstream, logically demonstrated weight reduction strategy known as the keto diet. At the point when you consolidate those intermittent fasting powers with the keto diet, you, truth be told, get the most forceful weight reduction.

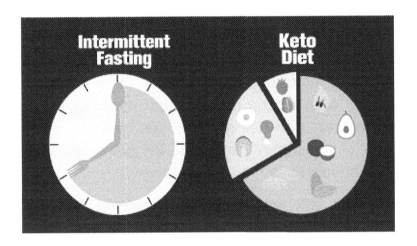

Both of these abstaining from excessive food intake plans are amazingly famous for various reasons. One of the primary reasons lies in the way that they bring various medical advantages as well as assisting with weight reduction progress. Before we get to those means you need to take toward fusing intermittent fasting into your way of life, we will talk about what intermittent fasting is, the thing that its advantages are and other significant snippets of data, so you can take a slow action towards this methodology.

It's critical that you make one stride at the time in assistance of creating your change as smooth as possible you have confidence that you have burned-through the perfect measures of supplements your body needs.

Truth be told, this is one of those objectives regardless of which consuming less calories plan you need to follow. You need to know every one of the significant realities before you really embrace your new abstaining from excessive food intake plan. As you do as such, you can make your eating fewer carbs progress totally smooth and you can make those progressions you will insight as could be expected. With this book, you will likewise study the significance of slimming down for both your physical and psychological well-being, you will realize what various sorts of consuming less calories plans are and their medical advantages.

Additionally, you will investigate how to benefit from intermittent fasting for boosting your weight reduction. The book likewise incorporates simple to follow, 30-day intermittent fasting difficulties which will assist you with accomplishing your ideal weight and lift your energy without battling.

As you investigate the book, you will, indeed, find a totally new, experimentally based way to deal with effortless weight reduction which can support your weight reduction venture as well as bring various other medical advantages your direction, which is something once in a while seen when following other eating fewer carbs plans.

You will investigate various ideas driving intermittent fasting; you will investigate various exercises on intermittent fasting which can bring about muscle acquire just as weight reduction.

With this book, you will likewise study distinctive intermittent fasting types which are presently overwhelming the whole wellness industry and substantially more which will help you draw nearer towards your weight and wellbeing objectives.

Exchanging." Keep as a primary concern that muscle versus fat is simply over the top food energy that has been put away; in the event that you keep on eating an overabundance, that abundance energy needs to discover some place to go, and muscle versus fat will keep on expanding. Then again, when you quick, your body goes to its own fat for a fuel source.

1.2 Fasting: A Historical Practice

As a custom, intermittent fasting is significantly more seasoned than the composed word. While utilizing it basically as a methods for weight reduction can be viewed as a moderately new wonder, it has a long history of utilization for things like heavenly correspondence, illness anticipation, improving fixation, diminishing the indications of maturing and then some. Fasting has been utilized by for all intents and purposes each religion and culture since the innovation of farming. Hippocrates, maybe the principal architect of current medication was rehearsing his exchange around 400 BC and quite possibly the most generally recommended medicines was of fasting routinely and drinking apple juice vinegar. He accepted (as it should be) that destroying takes fundamental assets through the stomach related cycle that the body could some way or another utilization for more beneficial cycles also. This thought came about in light of the fact that Hippocrates study the common tendency, everything being equal, to Ignore food while they are debilitated. Paracelsus, a contemporary of Hippocrates and the maker of the investigation of toxicology felt a similar way, venturing to such an extreme as to allude to the way toward fasting as the "doctor inside" in view of all the potential for great it can do in the human body. This inhabitant was afterward developed significantly more by in all honesty Benjamin Franklin who accepted that intermittent fasting was perhaps the most ideal approaches to fix a large group of normal illnesses. Strict works on; Fasting of some sort has consistently been seen by some as a profound practice which is likely why it is a significant inhabitant for religions all throughout the planet. Everybody from Buddha, to Muhammad, to Jesus Christ were completely known to lecture the advantages of fasting on a normal timetable. The Idea here is that the point of the training is to sanitize the physical or profound self, likely because of the increment in mental lucidity the interaction gives, with a scramble of its recuperating power tossed in just in case. Indeed, numerous Buddhists consistently eat in the first part of the day and afterward quick to the morning of the following day in request to feel considerably nearer to their confidence. Water diets that get longer and more as the expert ages are likewise very normal. With regards to Christianity, various groups quick for exacting time allotments for comparable reasons. The most limit illustration of this is maybe the Greek Orthodox Christians who quick for upwards of 200 days out of the year. Note that the Mediterranean Diet, which made it notable how solid individuals are around there, based quite a bit of it research in Crete which is generally Greek Orthodox. All things considered; It Is almost certain that intermittent fasting ought to be a characteristic piece of this eating routine also. In the biggest part of Christianity, Roman Catholicism, fasting Is conventional seen at a few central issues during that time and is for the most part rehearsed by eating one huge supper in the day just as two more modest dinners all at once that is near the main feast. This is most ordinarily seen on Ash Wednesday, which incorporates not eating any meat, and every one of the Fridays in the long stretch of Lent. While this isn't needed, it is mentioned by the individuals who are more established than 18 and under 59. This training as followed today is undeniably less exacting than it used to be preceding 1956. Other than nowadays, Roman Catholics are required to follow the occasion known by the name the Eucharistic Fast. This is the quick that should occur an hour before the time the expert realizes they will be taking mass. This time span used to stretch out between 12 am and the hour of Mass on Saturday however was abbreviated to where it doesn't give any genuine advantages but to get the body used to not eating. In the Bahai confidence, experts work on fasting every day for 12 hours during the period of March and they keep away from fluids notwithstanding food sources. Everybody in the confidence between the periods of IS and 70 is relied upon to take part on the off chance that they believe they can do it appropriately. Fasting is likewise consistently seen as a component of the Muslim confidence during Ramadan. This is a comparative light quick that even bars water. The prophet Muhammad was likewise referred to energize customary intermittent fasting also. Fasting is additionally a significant piece of the Hindu religion as it requests its supporters to notice a few distinct sorts from diets dependent on neighborhood custom and individual conviction. It is regular for some Hindus to quick certain days of every month. Moreover, the individual days of the week are additionally committed to fasting dependent on which god the expert is given to. The individuals who love Shiva commonly quick on Mondays, supporters of Vishnu keep an eye on quick on Thursdays and devotees of Ayyappa ordinarily quick on Saturdays. Fasting is additionally a typical piece of life in India where they consistently quick on explicit days. In numerous pieces of the country, they quick on Tuesdays in regard of the god called Lord Hanuman. This is a fluid just quick for the day however a few supporters will devour natural product also.

1.3 The Origin of Intermittent Fasting

Restorative fasting turned into a pattern during the 1800s as a method of forestalling or treating chronic weakness. Done under a specialist's oversight, this kind of fasting was embraced to get numerous conditions from hypertension migraines. Each quick was custom-made to the person's requirements. It very well may be only a day or as long as a quarter of a year.

In spite of the fact that fasting become undesirable as new prescriptions were created, it has as of late reappeared. In 2019, "intermittent fasting" was quite possibly the most ordinarily looked through terms. All in all, what would it be advisable for you to think about it?

1.4 Why is Intermittent Fasting Diet so popular?

Heftiness is turning into an expanding issue. Thus, it's no big surprise that such countless individuals are searching for a superior method to get more fit. Conventional weight control plans that confine calories frequently neglect to work for some individuals. It's hard to follow this sort of diet in the long haul. This frequently prompts yo-yo counting calories an interminable pattern of weight reduction and gain. Not exclusively does this frequently bring about emotional wellness issues, it can likewise prompt much more weight acquire generally.

It does not shock anyone, at that point, that numerous individuals have been looking for an eating regimen that can be kept up long haul. Intermittent fasting is one such eating routine. Even more a way of life change than an eating plan, it is unique in relation to ordinary eating regimens. Numerous supporters of intermittent fasting think that it's simple to follow for broadened periods. Far better, it assists them with getting more fit viably.

Nonetheless, this kind of eating plan additionally offers benefits past weight reduction. Numerous individuals accept that it can offer other wellbeing and health benefits as well. A portion of those advantages are even said to extend further some say it makes them more beneficial and centered. Thus, they can turn out to be more fruitful in the work environment. There have been late stories in the media of CEOs who guarantee their prosperity is all down to intermittent fasting.

However, the advantages don't stop there. There is some proof to show that intermittent fasting (or IF) helps health in alternate ways as well. It has been said to improve glucose levels and insusceptibility. It might support mind work, decline irritation and fix cells in the body as well.

In light of the entirety of this current, it's not difficult to perceive any reason why this method of eating is getting more well-known. Here, we'll investigate why intermittent fasting attempts to advance weight reduction. We'll look at the advantages of this way of life change and we'll tell you the best way to begin with this eating regimen convention.

1.5 How is Intermittent Fasting Different from Other Diet Plans?

Intermittent fasting (or IF for short) is a form of eating that occurs in lieu of a regular eating schedule. The focus in most eating plans is on the food you're eating. Weight watchers are restricted to a certain amount of calories or particular foods. Calorie counters will think about what they are and aren't allowed to eat as a result of this. Foods that are greasy or sweet are strictly forbidden. Vegetables, foods produced from the ground up, and low-sugar dinners are all getting a lot of attention. Many who practice these gobbling techniques often fantasies about sweets and bites. Though they may lose weight, they may struggle to stick to their diet in the long run.

Intermittent fasting is a one-of-a-kind practice. Rather than being a diet, it is a way of life. It involves eating plans that alternate between fasting and eating windows. It doesn't focus on the food you're consuming, unlike some other eating plans. When everything else is equal, it comes down to when you should feed. A few calorie counters enjoy the increased visibility this provides. They are free to consume the food sources that they enjoy. Many people even feel that it is more compatible with their lifestyles. In any case, there are certain possible pitfalls when it comes to using IF to lose weight.

1.6 The Most Popular Types of Intermittent Fasting Diet Plans

Intermittent fasting comes in a variety of forms. All has a distinct afterlife. Both adhere to the same standard of restricting food entry for a set period of time. Regardless, the amount of time between eating windows and the gap between them varies.

The 16:8 fast is perhaps the most well-known IF technique. This involves an 8-hour eating window followed by a 16-hour fast. Many people find this to be the most beneficial choice for them. They will easily incorporate skipping breakfast or supper into their daily routine.

Another famous IF choice is the 24-hour quick. This is now and then known as the Eat-Stop-Eat technique. It includes eating typically one day at that point staying away from nourishment for the accompanying 24 hours. The holes in the middle of diets could be just about as short as 24 hours or as long as 72 hours.

The 5:2 fasting technique is additionally mainstream. This includes eating typically for five days of the week. The other two back to back days, the weight watcher ought to limit their calorie utilization to around 500-600 calories.

A few IF weight watchers pick the 20:4 technique. This includes focusing all eating every day into a four-hour window. During the other 20 hours of the day, the weight watcher ought to eat no calories.

There are a few different sorts of fasting diet. A few group follow stretched out diets of up to 48 or 36 hours. Others quick for considerably more expanded periods. In case you're thinking about attempting IF, you'll need to pick the correct technique for you.

In comparison to other methods of calorie restriction, IF allows calorie counters to consume just as much as they need. They can eat whatever sweet or greasy foods they want. They won't have to worry about calorie counting when they go out to eat. They don't have to eat foods they despise. They don't have to feel as if they're depriving themselves of their favorite items. It's not difficult to see why this is such a common decision.

That, however intermittent fasting offers a lot a bigger number of advantages than different sorts of diet. Indeed, it advances quick weight reduction. Nonetheless, it likewise assists calorie counters with feeling more engaged and be more beneficial. It assists them with feeling better and more enthusiastic. With the health benefits that this method of eating brings, it's no big surprise individuals lean toward it to normal weight control plans.

1.8 The Basics of Intermittent Fasting Diet Plan

The act of intermittent fasting has been around for innumerable hundreds of years and utilized for almost as a wide range of purposes. Notwithstanding, the explanation that a great many people have caught wind of the training these days is on account of its demonstrated capacity to help the individuals who practice it get thinner and keep it off in the long haul while simultaneously feeling more empowered than they have In years. The most awesome thing? Getting into the intermittent fasting way of life doesn't expect you to surrender the food varieties you adore or even eat less calories per supper. Indeed, the most usually utilized sort of intermittent fasting makes it feasible for the individuals who practice it to skip breakfast prior to eating two suppers later in the day. This kind of way of life change is ideal for the individuals who wind up experiencing difficulty staying with a stricter eating routine arrangement as it doesn't take a very remarkable change to begin seeing genuine outcomes, instead of being compelled to change everything at the same time. Indeed, this is the thing that settles on intermittent fasting an extraordinary decision for both the long and present moment as it is simple enough to begin with and stay with in the long haul and furthermore viable enough to produce ceaseless outcomes so the individuals who practice it are persuaded to keep up their great work.

The explanation that intermittent fasting is so fruitful is a direct result of the Incontrovertible truth that your body carries on distinctively when it is in a taken care of state rather than when it is in a fasting state. A took care of state is any timeframe when your body is at present retaining supplements from food while processing it. This state begins around five minutes after you have completed your supper and will stay for upwards of five hours relying upon the kind of feast it was and how troublesome It Is for your body to separate It into energy. While your body is in this state It Is continually delivering insulin, which makes it definitely more hard for the body to consume fat than it is when insulin creation isn't occurring?

The following old happens straightforwardly following processing before the abstained state has happened. It is known as the cushion period and it will then last anyplace somewhere in the range of eight and 12 hours dependent on what you last ate and individual body science. It is just during this flat, when your Insulin levels have gotten back to typical that your body will actually want to consume fat at top effectiveness. Because of the measure of time needed to arrive at a genuine fasting record, numerous individuals never feel its NH impacts as they seldom go eight hours without eating, considerably less 12. This doesn't mean making the progress is unimaginable, in any case, you should simply guarantee you exploit this normal state as a method of breaking the three squares a day propensity.

You might be hearing a great deal about intermittent fasting as of late, yet it's not new. Indeed, one of the most seasoned known logical examinations on intermittent fasting goes back 75 years! Furthermore, the idea overall returns considerably further to the times of chasing and assembling regardless of whether your progenitors weren't doing it deliberately. Intermittent fasting has stood the trial of time since it isn't simply one more eating regimen. It's an amazing eating system that has significant impacts when done effectively. While intermittent fasting can unquestionably assist you with shedding pounds, its medical advantages go far past that. It can likewise expand your energy, improve your fixation, lessen puffiness and aggravation, and help shield you and your mind from different persistent sicknesses. There's some disarray encompassing intermittent fasting, however. A few group believe it's simply an extravagant method of limiting calories, yet it's far beyond that. In this part, you'll get familiar with the essentials of intermittent fasting and why it's so incredible. You'll likewise find the distinction between intermittent fasting and calorie limitation and why you should kick low-calorie diets to the control until the end of time.

1.9 Intermittent Fasting Diet Plan Benefits

The fasting state is ideal with regards to shedding pounds and building muscle, however these are just two of the essential advantages of intermittent fasting. Perhaps the most startling advantages for some, individuals is the measure of time you will wind up saving when you abruptly don't need to stress over eating a whole feast, particularly in the event that you take the customary course and cut out breakfast, saving urgent time in what Is regularly the most feverish piece of the day for some individuals. Along comparable lines, you will likewise find that you have additional cash in your food spending plan as breakfast food sources are frequently the absolute priciest also. The distinction will probably be recognizable, regardless of whether you eat somewhat more all through the remainder of the day too. While the Idea of surrendering a whole feast each day may appear to be incomprehensible now, with training you will be shocked at how sensible it will turn into. It will absolutely be great also in light of the fact that, as well as guaranteeing there is additional time in your day and additional cash in your ledger, it can straightforwardly help you live a more extended, better life. Truth be told, examines show that when you invest additional time in the abstained express your body redirects that energy to its center endurance frameworks similarly it would when you are starving. While your body may see them as the equivalent for the time being, the truth is that the two states are incredibly unique which implies that the final product is that your body winds up revived by the interaction instead of being supported.

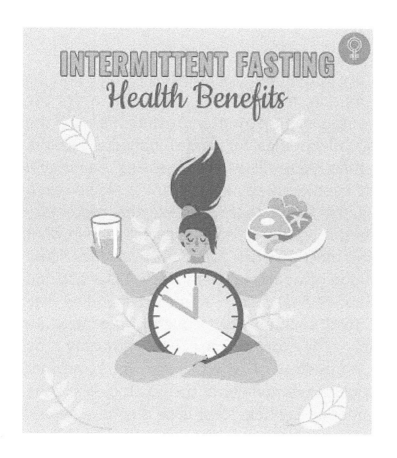

INTERMITTENT FASTING
Health Benefits

In particular, on the off chance that you invest a delayed time of energy in an abstained state you will enormously diminish your danger of stroke alongside your danger of a wide assortment of cardiovascular issues. It has additionally been demonstrated to decrease the impacts of chemotherapy in malignant growth patients too. Furthermore, these medical advantages don't require months or years to show up, they begin to arise when you start intermittent fasting and abatement your generally caloric admission by more than IS percent. Significantly more, benefits emerge as upgrades to regenerative organ and kidney work, circulatory strain, oxidative opposition and glucose resilience.

While all the 'Refined coarse with regards to why skirting a couple of suppers, every day prompts such emotional advantages isn't clear, what researchers have decided is that it is identified with the decrease of redundant pressure that the body encounters while fasting instead of eating three huge dinners daily. This is additionally why it improves the strength of the stomach related parcel just as that of numerous significant organs. It even gives the mitochondria in your body a lift, guaranteeing they use the energy accessible to them as productively as could really be expected. This, thus, has the additional gainful impact of diminishing the chances of oxidation harm happening anyplace in the framework.

The medical advantages to the body are eminent enough that both substitute days fasting, and numerous types of intermittent fasting are a medicinally affirmed method of diminishing one's danger of creating type 2 diabetes for the individuals who are now encountering the side effects of pre-diabetes. Presently, this advantage can absolutely be invalidated, which is the reason it is essential to not blame the way that you are fasting so as to feline everything and anything that you need, some restraint will in any case be required. This is the reason the most ideal decision is to not treat your time fasting as some extraordinary accomplishment, however to rather go about like it is only a normal piece of your daily practice. To see exactly how compelling intermittent fasting can be, consider a test that was performed on yeast cells that discovered when the yeast was denied of food its cells started to isolate all the more gradually accordingly. At the point when applied to your cells this means while you are fasting every one of your cells in a real sense lives longer than would some way or another be the case on account of this fake shortage. While the above rundown of medical advantages ought to be sufficient to in any event make the vast majority mull over Intermittent fasting prior to excusing it out and out, when they begin numerous individuals are amazed to And that something they appreciate most about the Intermittent fasting measure Is the way that it is a particularly basic yet gainful expansion to their day. It is so natural to use, truth be told, that in an investigation of those in excess of 30 pounds overweight, it was tracked down that more members had the option to adhere to an intermittent fasting plait than some other over a three-month timeframe. Additionally, while they were rehearsing intermittent fasting, this gathering of people saw a similar by and large measure of weight reduction as any other person. Maybe generally promising of all, in any case, Is that a year after the investigation had been finished, a greater amount of the individuals who had been intermittent fasting were as yet with it contrasted with the others and they had singularly lost the most weight by and large.

1.10 Getting started

With such countless advantages out there, you might be naturally restless to begin for yourself. To guarantee you can stay with the act of intermittent fasting as long as possible, nonetheless, there are a couple of rules you should remember. Buns more than you ear: While the Idea that you need to consume a bigger number of calories than you burn-through is a long way from progressive, it is particularly imperative to remember it while you are fasting irregularly as It can be far simpler to indulge post-quick than would some way or another be the situation, particularly when you are as yet becoming acclimated to the interaction.

In the event that you do slip, it very well may be not difficult to unnecessary the entirety of your diligent effort for the day with only a couple lost nibbles. There are 3,500 calories in a pound which implies that every week you need to consume at least 3,500 calories contrasted with what you devour in the event that you need to keep up your weight reduction consistently. While you may encounter a period where you are losing more than that as your body acclimates to the new way of eating, a consistent one pound seven days is the ideal sum as anything over that is unstainable In the long haul without at last putting your wellbeing in danger.

Continuously stay in charge: In request to utilize Intermittent fasting viably, it is essential that you have a suitable relationship with food directly from the beginning. On the off chance that you are the kind of individual who feels like certain food varieties, particularly their #1 food sources have a draw over them and your determination departs for good at the site of them then you may struggle beginning with intermittent fasting. Keep in mind, it is essential that you have the determination to go at least 12 hours without eating as any caloric admission will be sufficient to begin producing insulin and accordingly reset the clock. You should have the option to remove 500 calories from your eating routine, each day, to lose a pound seven days.

Suggestion: Download any wellness application to your cell phone it will help you gauge the number of calories you ought to burn-through consistently. While guaranteeing that you don't eat an excess of is a fundamental piece of the interaction, it is just a large portion of the fight as the other half is guaranteeing that you don't release yourself excessively long without eating. On the off chance that you expect to make intermittent fasting part of your life in the long-tens then it is imperative that you figure out how to add it to your life in a sound design as going excessively far one way or the other is simply going to prompt disappointment and possibly genuine wellbeing problems

Stick with it: When it comes to utilizing Intermittent fasting consistently, It is Important to discover the variety that turns out best for you and afterward subside into a drawn out everyday practice rather than beginning and halting routinely. While you make certain to see a few outcomes immediately, it will require about a month for your body to completely acclimate to the interaction which implies you should be focused on the reason and patient just as nothing occurs without any forethought.

While you make certain to get yourself incredibly eager, from the outset, after your body has realized when it can begin expecting calories you will find that your appetite pretty much gets back to business as usual. Besides, a month ought to be sufficient opportunity to begin seeing actual outcomes and indeed which ought to be sufficient to support your psychological grit considerably more. Then again, on the off chance that you quickly switch between strategies for intermittent fasting, or just use it for short blasts from time to time, at that point as opposed to upgrade your body's capacity to get more fit normally while additionally fabricating muscle, you will all things considered and it troublesome a lot of anything viably as your body will be In a consistent mess. All things considered, all weight reduction will stop as it attempts to cling to each and every calorie imaginable until it can sort out what on earth is going on. On the off chance that you really desire to see the kinds of results you are looking then the most ideal approach to guarantee this is the case is to discover one timetable of eating that works for you and afterward stay with it.

Converse with a medical care proficient: while the facts confirm that intermittent fasting assists individuals with getting thinner and fabricate muscle, notwithstanding a large group of different advantages, this doesn't mean it is naturally for everybody or that it doesn't book alongside some results too. First of all, when you first change to an intermittent fasting way of life you are probably going to encounter the runs, blockage or scenes of both for the initial fourteen days or so as your body acclimates to its new propensities. Moreover, it is imperative to be cautious in not allowing yourself to gorge adjust you have completed the process of fasting as this can prompt inner harm too. Notwithstanding how solid you intend to be; in any case, it is significant that you talk your arrangements over with either a dietitian or medical care proficient to guarantee you don't wind up unintentionally doing yourself more mischief than anything.

1.11 Women and Intermittent Fasting Diet Plans

While intermittent fasting is useful for the two people, men's bodies do take to the progress more effectively than ladies' bodies do. Accordingly, as a lady, on the off chance that you desire to make intermittent fasting a solid piece of your way of life then there are a couple of extra things you need to remember.

Numerous ladies who have attempted intermittent fasting recognize its various advantages. These incorporate decreased dangers of coronary illness, acquiring slender muscle, suggested glucose levels, diminished danger of persistent infections like disease and numerous others. Notwithstanding, alongside the great come hormonal changes inside their bodies that carry with them some different changes to a functioning way of life.

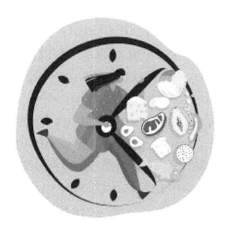

Nutrition deficiency: While embracing a intermittent fasting way of life, the main thing ladies need to remember is that the progress stage is likely going to interfere with the body's characteristic fruitfulness cycle. This is a protective component that is possibly disposed of when a satisfactory degree of sustenance Intake resumes. While fasting can influence your chemicals, intermittent fasting upholds legitimate hormonal equilibrium prompting a sound body and weight reduction the correct way once the body acclimates to the better approach for eating.

Additional challenges: While it isn't something that will influence everybody, a few ladies who routinely practice intermittent fasting do see issues like metabolic aggravations, beginning stage menopause, and missed periods. Likewise, on the off chance that you discover your body encountering delayed hormonal issues it could eventually prompt fair skin, balding, skin break out, diminished energy and the other, comparative issues. However long you don't take your fasting to the limit, at that point after the principal month or so you ought not to anticipate seeing any of these issues.

The explanation these hormonal Imbalances happen is that ladies are incredibly touchy to what exactly are known as starvation signals. All things considered, when a lady's body detects that it isn't accepting enough indispensable supplements it delivers a limit measure of the chemical's leptin and ghrelin to Increase the lady's longing to eat. All things considered, in the event that you find that you are totally eager when you arrive at the finish of your fasting stage then this could be the motivation behind why.

The explanation that ladies are quite a lot more helpless to this issue than men is to a great extent dependent on a protein called kisspeptin which is utilized by neurons to help in correspondence. It is additionally very touchy to ghrelin, leptin and insulin and present in far more noteworthy amounts in ladies than in men. At the point when the body produces exorbitant chemicals that quick you to eat, you are probably going to overlook them. Evidently, numerous ladies overlook these appetite signals, so the signs get much more Intense. The issue is that even these noisy signs are overlooked, and this may prompt gorging which can prompt the formation of a cycle that does little to guarantee your body gets the crucial supplements it needs while harming it in a larger number of ways than one. On the off chance that the negative propensities persevere for a really long time, it is conceivable that it can toss your chemicals messed up for all time.

Metabolism concerns: Your digestion Is Intimately attached to your wellbeing which implies that assuming you are encountering physiological or actual difficulties, your wellbeing could likewise be in danger. Fortunately, keeping a solid eating routine while working out, working out and fasting consistently would all be able to assist with settling these kinds of wellbeing challenges. Over the long haul, intermittent fasting has even appeared to assist offset with trip chemicals which implies you simply should know about the Issue and brave it while your body acclimates to your new propensities.

Protein concerns: Ladies will in general burn-through less protein contrasted with men. It follows then that fasting ladies devour even less protein. Less utilization of protein brings about less amino acids in the body. Amino acids are fundamental for the union of insulin-like development factor in the liver which initiates estrogen receptors. The development factor IGF-1 causes the uterine divider covering to thicken just as the movement of the conceptive cycle.

A delayed low protein admission can likewise influence your estrogen levels, which can likewise influence your metabolic capacity and the other way around. This can possibly influence your temperament, processing, insight, bone arrangement and that's only the tip of the iceberg. It can even influence the mind as estrogen is needed to invigorate the neurons liable for stopping the creation of the synthetics that direct hunger. Basically, any time your estrogen levels drop recognizably you are probably going to wind up feeling hungrier than would somehow or another be the situation.

As recently examined, ladies are normally more delicate to sensations of appetite than men are which is the reason numerous ladies find that fasting can be such a test. Fortunately, there is a variety of intermittent fasting that has been intended to locally available ladies all the more effectively into an intermittent fasting way of life. It is known as Crescendo Fasting and to follow it, you should simply begin by fasting three days every week on nonconsecutive days. You will find that you actually see a large number of the general advantages of intermittent fasting, without exposing yourself to the potential for hormonal awkwardness. This methodology is far gentler on the body during the progress time frame and it can assist you with changing fasting as fast as could really be expected. Assuming you still and that you are having issues, you can begin your day with around 250 calories prior to continuing to proceed with your quick as should be expected.

Advantages: The advantages of this style of intermittent fasting are for the most part In accordance with what the more thorough variants gloat and include:

• You acquire energy

• Improving provocative markers

• Losing weight and muscle versus fat

• No hormonal difficulties

Crescendo fasting Rules:

Above all, it is important that you do not fast for more than three days a week during the main month and never for more than 24 hours at a time. During these fasting times, you will need to fast for somewhere between 12 and 16 hours; it is important that you do not fast for more than 16 hours at a time if at all possible. When you do fast, you'll always need to work out, so do something light or wait until after you've broken your quick to start. While you are fasting, you are still allowed to drink water. As long as you don't add something calorie-dense to your espresso or tea, you're good to go. If you think you'll be close to the 16-hour mark, you may want to add some coconut oil and grass-fed margarine to your espresso. This approach to fasting informs your body that it is the perfect time for your cells to eat fat in order to obtain energy and clean up their act. For women, crescendo fasting has a distinct benefit. It will also contribute to your wealth and appeal. After two or three weeks, you will notice the benefits that come with it.

- Radiant skin

- Healthy moxie

- Shiny hair

- A lively attitude

- Appropriate body weight

On the off chance that you are beyond 90 a few years old, in excess of a couple of pounds overweight, at that point you should consider adding grass-took care of collagen to your espresso on your fasting days all things being equal. Collagen can reset your leptin levels which will help battle hunger. During fasting days it is critical to keep both your fructose and sugars levels to a base as this will assist with advancing leptin levels in the body.

Chapter 2: The Importance of Nutrition

You're day by day abstaining from excessive food intake decisions unquestionably have a huge effect with regards to your actual wellbeing as well as to your emotional wellness state. Individuals are typically mindful of the way that having great nourishment and participating in actual work can help them keep up that ideal weight, yet in addition keep up their general wellbeing.

All things considered, truly the significance and advantages of having great nourishment and following a solid counting calories plan go a long ways past keeping up that ideal weight. Truly the food varieties you eat bring numerous other medical advantages, for example, diminishing the danger of building up certain sicknesses like diabetes, stroke, coronary illness, osteoporosis, a few malignant growths and others.

The food varieties you eat likewise can assist with the decrease of hypertension, they can help you lower elevated cholesterol levels, assist you with improving your general prosperity, improve your capacity to ward off various types of sicknesses, improve your capacity to recuperate from wounds and illness just as help you increment your energy levels.

2.1 What is Nutrition?

Nourishment likewise is known as sustenance. Sustenance is viewed to as the stockpile of various materials or food sources which are needed by the body and the body's cells instead of creating and stay alive.

In human medication and science, nourishment is viewed as the training or study of using and burning-through food varieties. Likewise, in clinical focuses and medical clinics, nourishment additionally may allude to the specific patients' food prerequisites including distinctive healthful arrangements which are conveyed by means of intra gastric cylinders or through intravenous.

In all actuality the human body requires a few significant nourishment types for improvement, development and remaining alive. There are additionally some pivotal supplements which don't furnish the body with energy, yet they are still critical like fiber and water, notwithstanding macronutrients for remaining alive.

With regards to macronutrients, they are critical, as without devouring them, it is difficult to work. Notwithstanding macronutrients the body needs, we likewise need different arrangements, for example, minerals and nutrients which are additionally urgent natural mixtures.

As hereditary qualities advance, organic chemistry and sub-atomic science, just as sustenance definitely have gotten an ever increasing number of zeroed in on various metabolic pathways digestion all in all. Nourishment clarifies diverse biochemical strides, through which various arrangements or substances inside the body are being changed, utilized as fuel sources.

Nourishment as a science is likewise committed to clarifying how unique medical problems and distinctive ailments can be decreased or even forestalled with great sustenance and sound consuming less calories draws near. Along these lines, nourishment likewise includes assessments on how unique ailments and infections can be brought about by certain dietary factors like food sensitivities, unhealthiness brought about by a horrible eating routine just as various food prejudices.

Appropriately, nourishment is viewed as the admission of various food varieties corresponding to the human body's dietary requirements. Hence, great sustenance is viewed as a sound and sufficient just as a reasonable eating fewer carbs plan which when joined with a standard exercise approach brings about great wellbeing.

Then again, helpless abstaining from excessive food intake decisions can prompt expanded defenselessness to various types of infections, diminished invulnerability, and hindered both mental and actual advancement just as extraordinarily decreased efficiency.

It can likewise be said that nourishment is the cycle by which people devoured and used diverse food substances in any case; those fundamental supplements which incorporate fat, protein, carbs, nutrients, electrolytes and minerals.

Around the vast majority of our everyday energy use comes from carbs and fats while around fifteen percent of our day by day energy use comes from burned-through proteins.

In people, nourishment is accomplished through the critical cycle of burning-through food varieties. With regards to the necessary measures of those fundamental supplements, these vary starting with one individual then onto the next relying upon their age, their condition of the body like their active work, meds taken and other clinical components.

2.2 What is Good Nutrition?

As recently referenced, great nourishment is unquestionably the main factor with regards to keeping up both great physical and psychological wellness states.

Indeed, eating an even eating routine is an urgent piece of having great wellbeing for each individual regardless of their age, ailments and different variables which vary starting with one individual then onto the next.

Sustenance as the examination or the study of various supplements contained in food varieties we burn-through, likewise shows us how the body really utilizes these various supplements just as shows us the connection between infection, wellbeing, and our consuming less calories decisions.

In the event that your nourishment is acceptable, it implies that you burn-through every one of those fundamental supplements your body needs for working at its best levels.

In the event that your consuming less calories decisions are acceptable, you shield yourself from different sorts of ailments and infections like coronary illness, heftiness, stroke, malignancy, diabetes, and numerous others.

Sadly, today numerous individuals rotate their slimming down decisions around immersed fats, sugars, or trans fats just as more sodium-stuffed vegetables and organic products. With these helpless counting calories decisions, the body's wellbeing may decay as it considers what we devour each day.

Settling on helpless slimming down decisions, indeed, decreases by and large prosperity, causes various issues with weight, for example, weight gain or weight reduction, harms the safe framework, makes us drained and fomented.

Helpless counting calories decisions additionally accelerate those maturing impacts, increment the dangers of building up certain illnesses, and contrarily influences the state of mind, diminishes both concentration and efficiency and numerous other amazingly adverse consequences.

As should be obvious, those food decisions you make each day altogether influence your general wellbeing, influencing how you will feel today, how you will tomorrow and how you will feel later on. Therefore, having a decent, even eating regimen is quite possibly the most vital advances prompting having a better way of life.

Actually an even eating regimen, when joined with a normal active work of any sort, can help you draw nearer towards your ideal weight, assist you with keeping up your ideal load just as decrease your dangers of creating diverse ailments.

2.3 Calculating your Body Mass Index

As recently expressed in the book, nourishment is critical for both turn of events and development just as for generally prosperity and by and large wellbeing.

Eating an even eating routine to just contributes emphatically to your physical and psychological wellness state, yet in addition adds to forestalling sicknesses prompting gigantic enhancements in your day to day existence quality and your life expectancy. With regards to your wholesome status, it is viewed as your general condition of wellbeing dictated by the food varieties you eat.

There are a few unique ways with regards to evaluating your generally speaking dietary situations with as your everyday food admission, your biochemical estimations, and your actual body estimations or your anthropometric estimations.

One of those vital markers of your overall nourishing status is your BMI or your weight list. Your BMI considers your tallness and your weight just as corresponds with the aggregate sum of fat you have, which is for this situation communicated as a specific level of your body weight.

It ought to be noticed that the genuine connection communicated in BMI details rely upon age following the most noteworthy relationship was found in people of ages between 26 and 55 years while the least relationship is found in the older populace.

To compute your BMI status or your weight record, you need to take your weight communicated in kilograms and separation it by your stature communicated in meters squared. That number you get communicates your weight list. It ought to be noticed that those higher qualities show more noteworthy fat stores entire those lower number demonstrate deficient stores of fat.

When you have your weight list decided, it tends to be exceptionally useful filling in as your own analytic device whether you are underweight or overweight.

On the off chance that your weight list number if somewhere in the range of 25 and 29, you are overweight while a weight record number which is over 3o arranges as fat.

You should press towards having a solid weight record which is somewhere in the range of 18.5 and 24.9. As well as deciding your general nourishment status, weight record likewise computes the measure of fat contained in the body which is particularly significant for competitors, ladies who are pregnant and jocks.

Weight list generally speaking overestimates the fat sum in the body for these gatherings while it belittles the fat contained in the body in old individuals just as in people who battle with some sort of actual incapacity, who have issues with their muscles or who can't walk.

It ought to be noticed that that in spite of these advantages weight list isn't the absolute best proportion of wellbeing and weight hazard as there is likewise an abdomen condition which should be considered with regards to foreseeing wellbeing chances.

In addition, that wellbeing weight record scope of 20 to 25 is just appropriate for grown-ups and not for kids. Truth be told, for grown-up individuals who have quit creating and growing, an increment in their weight list is most much of the time brought about by a critical expansion in their muscle to fat ratio.

Then again, kids who are as yet during the time spent developing and creating, their fat sum in the body changes after some time which likewise causes changes in their weight record.

Consequently, weight list diminishes during those preschool years while it will in general increment as we enter adulthood. Consequently, a weight list for youths and kids should be looked at considering their age just as their sexual orientation outlines.

2.4 Calculating your Waist Circumference

As referenced in the past part of the book, another extraordinary apparatus you can use for deciding your wellbeing chances, as well as utilizing your weight list, is your abdomen perimeter.

Truth be told, your midsection outline is a far superior wellbeing hazard indicator than simply weight list. Truly having a potbelly or having fat around your midsection regardless of your real size brings more wellbeing chances, particularly for those stoutness related ailments.

Truth be told, fat which is predominately arranged around the midsection is more perilous than fat which is arranged around the rump and hips. There are various investigations directed on the subject which recommend that the appropriation of those fat sources is related with various wellbeing dangers, for example, having more elevated cholesterol levels, creating heart illnesses or diabetes.

Lesser wellbeing chances are identified with having no potbelly or being thin around here while moderate danger is identified with being overweight, however having no potbelly. The more serious danger from moderate to high danger is identified with being thin, however having a potbelly and high danger is identified with being overweight and having a potbelly.

Since abdomen outline is identified with a wide range of wellbeing chances, it is a smart thought that you measure your midsection. For men, having at least 94 centimeters in the midsection shows an expanded danger while having at least 102 in centimeters around the midriff demonstrates a generously expanded wellbeing hazard.

The numbers are somewhat less for ladies. Having at least eight centimeters around the midsection for ladies shows a marginally expanded danger while having 88 centimeters around the abdomen demonstrates a considerably expanded danger.

It ought to be noticed that accepting standard actual work, keeping away from undesirable propensities, for example, smoking and burning-through more unsaturated fats rather soaked fats can diminish the danger of creating issues related with stomach weight.

2.5 Why is Nutrition Important?

The effect of the eating fewer carbs decisions you make each day add to various spaces of your general wellbeing influencing both your physical and psychological wellness state. Truth be told, there have been various examinations directed on the point which propose that undesirable eating less junk food decisions have altogether added to the huge heftiness scourge in the US.

A similar report likewise recommended that around 33% of grown-ups in the United States, which is in excess of about a third of grown-up residents, are battling with corpulence. The numbers are not extraordinary for kids and young people either, as a similar report has proposed that in excess of seventeen millions youths and offspring of ages two to nineteen are likewise large.

Besides, even those people who have a sound weight additionally can battle with various ailments having some significant dangers which can cause diseases and sometimes even passing. These incorporate creating type 2 diabetes, having hypertension or hypertension, battling with osteoporosis or in any event, building up certain sorts of malignant growth.

Subsequently, it is critical that you center around changing your unfortunate eating designs by settling on keen decisions rotating around your eating regimen, you, truth be told, can shield yourself from various medical problems.

There are some other danger factors identified with helpless counting calories decisions like the advancement of certain sorts of persistent infection, which are lamentably progressively seen in grown-ups as well as in kids and youths of more youthful ages.

Truly the dietary propensities we have set up in our adolescence frequently keep during our adulthood years. Therefore, it is critical that guardians give time to showing their kids great nourishment, and how to eat quality food varieties. Truth be told, that connection between having great nourishment and having great weight altogether lessens the danger of building up those sorts of constant sicknesses; it is excessively significant for us to disregard it.

Therefore, it is critical to you find certain ways to accept a better, even eating routine which will help you fuel your body with the entirety of the significant supplements your body needs for working at its best, remaining solid, dynamic and sound.

Furthermore, very much like with expanding your actual work and accepting other sound propensities, rolling out these little improvements in your counting calories example can lead you far. At the point when you embrace an even eating regimen loaded with entire grains, vegetables, and organic products, you fulfill your craving levels as well as you simultaneously feed your general body.

Despite the fact that it is totally fine to enjoy some less quality food sources occasionally, it is critical that you're eating routine incorporates those fundamental supplements your body needs for endeavoring.

2.6 Benefits of Good Nutrition

In this part of the book, we will talk about additional a portion of the fundamental advantages of settling on great dietary decisions. One of them is that acceptable sustenance can essentially improve your general prosperity. Very much like eating less nutritious food sources diminishes both your psychological and actual wellbeing, people who devour food sources wealthy in supplements are less inclined to report having issues with their psychological and actual wellbeing.

Since eating permits us to be more dynamic as we have more energy, around 66% of people who routinely burn-through new vegetables and new natural products report no serious issues with their general wellbeing state. This is simple contrasted with those people who have some sort of emotional well-being problem who by and large have a terrible eating routine, and eat less nutritious food varieties.

In compatibility of securing your general prosperity and your general wellbeing state, your food decisions ought to incorporate those fundamental supplements which will be talked about in the following segment of the book.

Settling on the correct slimming down decisions additionally forestalls the advancement of different sicknesses. Indeed, having great nourishment and even dietary patterns can decrease your danger of building up certain sorts of coronary illness, type 2 diabetes or having hypertension and raised cholesterol levels.

Normally, keeping up great nourishment additionally assists you with remaining in the correct shape, assisting you with the upkeep of your ideal weight. Eating normal food sources rather than handled food sources decidedly impacts your weight just as your general wellbeing state.

In actuality, being overweight builds your dangers for creating ongoing conditions, for example, type 2 diabetes, which when left untreated, can restrict your versatility while harming your joints. Thus, toward remaining fit as a fiddle, you're eating routine ought to incorporate a lot of entire grains, vegetables, products of the soil food sources wealthy in fundamental supplements.

Truth be told, keeping an even eating regimen notwithstanding standard actual work is the best way to get thinner and keep up it over the long haul. There is no supernatural pill or enchanted beverage which may assist people with losing those extra pounds. There are just acceptable sustenance and an expansion in actual work as the regular method of shedding pounds.

Individuals regularly battle with famous eating less junk food plans as they for the most part confine their #1 food varieties. This can work in the short run as people for the most part embrace their old eating fewer carbs propensities for quite a while. Toward staying away from this issue, the best thought is to rethink those old plans, add a few tones with those new veggies, and mix it up.

It is likewise critical to treat yourself for certain less good food sources now and again as everything is about balance. It isn't tied in with confining yourself from those food sources you appreciate, however it is tied in with adding some more to them. Truth be told, adding new veggies and organic products can have an immense effect assisting you with controlling your cholesterol levels, and your circulatory strain just as your weight.

This is actually where intermittent fasting goes to the game. Rather than fixating on your day by day calorie admission, rather than eating food varieties that you abhor, you figure out how to change your present consuming less calories examples and spotlight on when you eat rather than what you eat. Today it is incredibly costly to be undesirable. In all actuality individuals battling with consuming less calories decisions are bound to build up some sort of ailments because of their helpless eating fewer carbs decisions and being debilitated accompanies costs.

Thus, there is nothing unexpected in the way that in excess of over two thirds of the medical care and clinical consideration dollars in the United States are spent on treating preventable illnesses identified with consuming less calories decisions. You likely have encountered eating a lot of food varieties and out of nowhere getting a charge out of an explosion of energy just to feel totally depleted in an exceptionally brief timeframe later.

This happens in light of the fact that the body responds upon those food sources containing countless refined sugars. In expanding energy levels which will last subsequent to devouring food varieties, you need to stay away from unfortunate food sources and spotlight on burning-through food varieties which are loaded with fundamental supplements your body will use as its fuel.

As you embrace great eating less junk food decisions, you can at long last build your energy levels which will last for the duration of the day, not for only a few hours and in particular, you won't encounter those standard fail spectacularly impacts.

Besides, you will actually want to zero in additional on what's going on around you, which isn't the situation when you feel depleted and tired. As you most likely are aware, the body gets energy from those food varieties we ingest just as from fluids we devour.

The fundamental supplements the body utilizes as its energy powers are protein, fats, and carbs. Those carbs like entire grains, boring vegetables, and bread are the best fuel sources since they are processed much slowly.

Additionally, water is likewise one of those fundamental components vital for supplement transportation.

Lick of water or parchedness can prompt absence of energy, so as much it is critical to burn-through those fundamental supplements, it is additionally essential to keep your body hydrated. Furthermore, an iron inadequacy can likewise cause low energy levels and peevishness just as weariness. Hence, you're eating regimen ought to likewise remember food varieties rich for iron; verdant veggies like spinach, peas, and poultry just as fish.

In compatibility of acquiring the most from these food sources, the best thought is to build your nutrient C admission simultaneously. Consider adding a greater amount of those nutrient C-rich food sources like verdant greens, broccoli, tomatoes, kiwi and peppers.

Great sustenance likewise assists with keeping your invulnerable framework working at its best. As you probably are aware, our insusceptible framework helps us battling ailments and sicknesses, and yet, having helpless sustenance implies your resistant framework is harmed, so it can't work as expected.

For keeping up your resistant framework, your body requires a specific admission of those fundamental supplements just as legitimate minerals and nutrients. Henceforth, eating an even eating routine loaded with those supplements can help you support your resistant framework.

Great nourishment additionally can assist with your skin wellbeing just as help you postpone maturing impacts. Eating an even eating routine not just influences your energy levels, your safe framework, and your weight yet in addition assumes a pivotal part with regards to your skin wellbeing.

As per the most recent examinations directed on the theme, food sources which are plentiful in nutrient E and C, wealthy in cell reinforcements and lycopene help additionally help shield your skin from sun harm. Food varieties like nuts, avocados, berries, tomatoes, and fish all come loaded with fundamental minerals and supplements which are astounding for the skin.

For example, tomatoes are loaded with nutrient C that helps in the structure of collagen that improves the skin, firmer and smoother which postpones maturing impacts. What's more, berries are additionally extraordinary for the skin as they are loaded with nutrients and cell reinforcements which advance skin recovery keeping your skin smooth, firm and new.

As referenced already, accepting a decent eating regimen likewise implies you decrease your danger of building up certain sorts of persistent infections, for example, hypertension, type a diabetes and other.

These danger factors are fundamentally expanded in people who are overweight or who eat horribly. In feet, among grown-up people between ages reason for visual deficiency, kidney disappointment, and amazingly removal.

Burning-through good food sources can decidedly influence your mind-set just as your generally speaking emotional well-being state. Consuming less calories plans which are limited in starches admission normally increment those pressure sentiments while eating less junk food plans which advance carbs accompany considerably more inspiring impacts influencing mind-set.

Likewise, eating less junk food plans which are wealthy in proteins, low in fat and moderate in carbs additionally have significantly constructive outcomes on emotional well-being and state of mind since they give the body sufficient omega 3-unsaturated fats and iron supplies.

Similarly as the food varieties we burn-through influence our disposition, the state of mind can likewise influence our dietary decisions. At the point when we are tragic, we are bound to settle on undesirable dietary decisions while individuals who are more joyful are bound to pick better food sources.

Great nourishment, notwithstanding these medical advantages, additionally assists us with expanding our efficiency and core interest. Truly the food sources we devour hugely affect the manner in which we feel and think. For example, when your body is coming up short on glucose, you are less inclined to think and center, as the cerebrum isn't accepting sufficient energy.

Counting calories plans which are extremely high in cholesterol and fat, indeed, can seriously harm the cerebrum by building plaque sources inside mind vessels which further harm the tissues of the cerebrum.

Thus, you ought to keep away from food varieties loaded with outrageous measures of fat and spotlight on eating more veggies and organic products which will help you remain on track and beneficial for the duration of the day.

Another stunning medical advantage of good sustenance is that it can stretch your life. As you most likely are aware, the body needs food varieties and supplements for developing, creating and enduring. Then again, the way toward separating food supplements, the way toward processing them, can make an enormous pressure the body.

Consequently, indulging makes more pressure the body which can cause a more limited life expectancy. As indicated by the most recent investigation directed on the theme, around eighteen percent of passing among American residents are added to stoutness.

In this way, being corpulent can prompt a huge decrease in by and large future in the United States as well as when all is said in done. The best thought is to accept dietary decisions which are loaded with fundamental supplements and stay away from handled food sources which cause more pressure to the body.

As you can see from this section, your dietary decisions influence your stomach as well as influence each organ in the body including your skin, mind, your heart, resistant framework and all the other things. Consequently, great sustenance can bring various medical advantages to ensuring and aiding you on a wide range of levels while expanding the general nature of your life.

Conclusion

Intermittent fasting can be done in a variety of ways, but they all revolve around choosing daily eating and fasting times. For example, you might try eating just for eight hours a day and fasting for the rest of the day. Alternatively, you might opt to eat just one meal a day two days a week. There are a variety of intermittent fasting schedules to choose from.

After many hours without food, the body's sugar reserves are depleted, and it begins to burn fat. This is referred to as metabolic switching by him. Intermittent fasting is in contrast to the typical eating style of most Americans, who feed continuously during the day. If anyone eats three meals a day plus snacks and does not exercise, they are consuming calories rather than burning fat stores every time they eat.

Intermittent fasting works by extending the time between when your body burns off the calories from your last meal and starts burning fat.

Before beginning intermittent fasting, make sure to consult your doctor. The actual procedure is easy once you have his or her permission. You can choose a regular approach, which limits daily eating to one six- to eight-hour span. For example, you might try 16/8 fasting, which involves eating for eight hours and fasting for sixteen. Most people find it easy to maintain this pattern over time.

INTERMITTENT

FASTING

DIET PLAN

A Beginners guide to Intermittent Fasting Step-By-Step.

Chapter 1. Intermittent Fasting induces Anticancer Serum

Metabolic condition is portrayed by focal weight, insulin opposition, raised circulatory strain, and dyslipidemia. Metabolic disorder is a huge danger factor for a few regular tumors (e.g., liver, colorectal, bosom, pancreas). Pharmacologic therapies utilized for the parts of the metabolic disorder seem, by all accounts, to be deficient to control malignancy improvement in subjects with metabolic condition. Murine models showed that malignant growth has the slowest movement when there is no food utilization during the day by day action stage. Intermittent fasting from sunrise to nightfall is a type of fasting working on during human movement hours. To test the anticancer impact of intermittent fasting from sunrise to dusk in metabolic disorder, we directed a pilot concentrate in 14 subjects with metabolic condition who abstained (no eating or drinking) from day break to nightfall for in excess of 14 h every day for four sequential weeks. We gathered serum tests before 4-week intermittent fasting, toward the finish of fourth week during 4-week intermittent fasting and 1 after quite a while following 4-week intermittent fasting. We performed serum proteomic examination utilizing Nano super elite fluid chromatography-pair mass spectrometry.

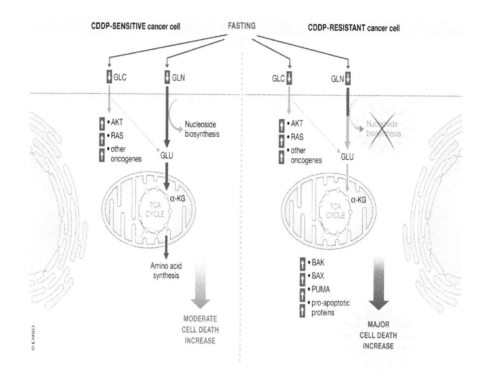

We tracked down a huge overlay expansion in the levels of a few tumor silencer and DNA fix quality protein items (GP) toward the finish of fourth week during 4-week intermittent fasting (CALU, INTS6, KIT, CROCC, PIGR), and 1 after a long time following 4-week intermittent fasting (CALU, CALR, IGFBP4, SEMA4B) contrasted and the levels before 4-week intermittent fasting. We additionally tracked down a critical decrease in the degrees of tumor advertiser GPs toward the finish of fourth week during 4-week intermittent fasting (POLK, CD109, CAMP, NIFK, SRGN), and 1 after a long time following 4-week intermittent fasting (CAMP, PLAC1) contrasted and the levels before 4-week intermittent fasting. Fasting from sunrise to nightfall for about a month additionally initiated an enemy of diabetes proteome reaction by up controlling the key administrative proteins of insulin motioning toward the finish of fourth week during 4-week intermittent fasting (VPS8, POLRMT, IGFBP-5) and 1 after a long time following 4-week intermittent fasting (PRKCSH), and an enemy of maturing proteome reaction by up managing H2B histone proteins 1 after a long time following 4-week intermittent fasting. Subjects had a huge decrease in weight record, abdomen perimeter, and improvement in pulse that co-happened with the anticancer, against diabetes, and hostile to maturing serum proteome reaction. These discoveries propose that intermittent fasting from sunrise to nightfall effectively adjusts the separate qualities and can be an assistant treatment in metabolic condition. Further examinations are expected to test the intermittent fasting from sunrise to dusk in the avoidance and therapy of metabolic disorder prompted diseases.

1.1 Introduction

One of the terrific difficulties of our occasions is the rising pervasiveness of metabolic condition. Metabolic condition is portrayed by focal weight, insulin opposition, raised circulatory strain, high fatty oil, and low high-thickness lipoprotein levels. Metabolic disorder has antagonistically affected numerous parts of society. Critically, metabolic condition is a huge danger factor for a few basic tumors (e.g., liver, colorectal, bosom, endometrium, and pancreas).

Disturbed circadian clock musicality has been perceived as one of the reasons for metabolic disorder and metabolic condition instigated malignancies. Pharmacologic therapies utilized for the segments of the metabolic disorder have all the earmarks of being lacking to decrease the danger of creating metabolic condition incited tumors. In addition, pharmacologic therapies can't reset the circadian clock musicality; consequently, there is a critical requirement for a successful mediation to reset the circadian clock and forestall metabolic condition and metabolic disorder initiated malignant growths. Creature examines showed that resetting the circadian clock by time-limited taking care of improves metabolic condition and restrains the advancement of disease. In this way, resetting the disturbed circadian check in people by sequential every day intermittent fasting could give an essential system to improve metabolic disorder and diminish the frequency of metabolic condition incited malignant growth. Fasting during movement hours rather than the latency hours of the day has all the earmarks of being significant for the streamlining of anticancer impact and quality articulation. Subject with no admittance to food during the action stage (dim period) of a 12-h light/12-h dim cycle had an essentially more slow tumor movement and higher endurance contrasted and subject that had no admittance to food during the dormancy stage (light stage), and subject that approached food not indispensable. Reliable with these discoveries, a previous murine examination showed that the uncoupling of the fringe timekeepers from the control of the focal clock possibly happened when subject had no admittance to food during the dynamic stage. Conversely, an insignificant change in the period of quality articulation was seen when subject had no admittance to food during the idle stage, relating to evening time in people. The discoveries of murine examinations ought to be deciphered with regards to the way that people are diurnal (action happens during daytime), and subject are nighttime (movement happens during evening time). The discoveries of these murine examinations are as per the discoveries of our starter contemplates directed in solid subjects. Our outcomes showed that 30-day intermittent fasting from day break to nightfall, the human movement stage, was related with an anticancer serum proteome reaction and up controlled a few key administrative proteins that assume a vital part in tumor concealment, DNA fix, insulin flagging, glucose, and lipid digestion, circadian clock, cytoskeletal redesigning, safe framework, and psychological capacity. Critically, the expansion in the levels of these basic administrative proteins happened without any huge weight reduction and calorie limitation. A few human examinations showed valuable impacts of intermittent fasting (e.g., Ramadan fasting, and time-confined eating in subjects with metabolic condition. Be that as it may, in none of these investigations, proteomic profiling was performed to comprehend the component behind the anticancer impact of intermittent fasting and time-confined eating in subjects with metabolic disorder.

To this end, we guessed that intermittent fasting from sunrise to nightfall rehearsed solely during the human movement hours for about a month would be related with an anticancer serum proteome reaction, up manage anticancer proteins and administrative proteins of DNA fix and insulin flagging, and down direct favorable to malignant growth proteins.

1.2 Methods

Study of Subjects

All exploration was directed as per significant rules and guidelines after composed educated assent was gotten from all subjects. The examination didn't fit the bill for imminent enrollment as a clinical preliminary in light of the fact that there was no investigation coordinated intercession. The strict quick was ongoing individual lead, not examination coordinated, and accordingly, the investigation was observational in examination plan. Consideration measures were as per the following: (1) Subjects who are 18 years of age or more seasoned; (2) Subjects who intend to quick during the strict month of Ramadan; (3) Subjects should meet any three of the accompanying five standards for metabolic condition as portrayed by Grundy et al.2 (a) focal weight surveyed by midriff circuit equivalent to or more prominent than 102 cm (40 inches) in men, and equivalent or more noteworthy than 88 cm (35 inches) in ladies; (b) fasting serum fatty oil level equivalent to or more prominent than 150 mg/dL or on drug treatment for hypertriglyceridemia (e.g., fibrates, nicotinic corrosive); (c) low high-thickness lipoprotein level under 40 mg/dL in men and under 50 mg/dL in ladies or on drug treatment for low high-thickness lipoprotein level (fibrates, nicotinic corrosive); (d) raised systolic circulatory strain equivalent to or more prominent than 130 or raised diastolic pulse equivalent to or more noteworthy than 85 or on drug treatment for hypertension, (e) raised fasting glucose level equivalent to or more noteworthy than 100 mg/dL or on drug treatment for hyperglycemia/diabetes); (4) Subjects who consented to go through Fibro Scan testing for assessment of hepatic steatosis and fibrosis. Subjects were avoided on the off chance that they had any of the accompanying: (1) powerlessness to give educated assent; (2) ladies who are pregnant or breastfeeding; (3) dynamic disease; (4) dynamic contamination requiring anti-microbial use; (5) seizure problem; (6) cardiovascular occasion during the most recent a half year; (7) utilization of liquor or sporting substances.

The essential result of this pilot study was the enlistment of an anticancer proteome reaction toward the finish of fourth week during 4-week intermittent fasting and 1 after a long time following 4-week intermittent fasting. The auxiliary results were improvement in the parts of metabolic condition, lipid board (absolute cholesterol, fatty substance, high-thickness lipoprotein, and low-thickness lipoprotein), hepatic board (egg whites, all out protein, alanine aminotransferase, aspartate aminotransferase, soluble phosphatase), and adiposity, oxidative pressure, and irritation biomarkers.

Study of Procedures

Subjects were booked for a screening visit inside three weeks of commencement of 4-week intermittent fasting at research facility. During this visit, their qualification was surveyed dependent on consideration and prohibition measures, and composed educated assent was taken. Clinical history and actual assessment were performed. Pulse estimations were performed very still and sitting position. A pee pregnancy test for the female subjects at childbearing age was performed. Hepatic steatosis and fibrosis were evaluated utilizing Fibro Scan with a controlled lessening boundary (CAP).

Subjects began fasting at sunrise after a pre-first light breakfast and finished fasting at nightfall (sunset) with a supper for 29 successive days. Severe fasting happened without eating or drinking among day break and nightfall (sunset), which are even change time regions of the day. There was no interventional calorie or energy limitation in any case. Subjects had their fundamental suppers at the change time regions of the day, including pre-sunrise breakfast (at the primary progress time) and supper at dusk (at the subsequent progress time) and were permitted to eat (e.g., bites) or drink on the off chance that they required among nightfall and first light notwithstanding the pre-sunrise breakfast and supper at dusk.

Information on weight, midsection perimeter and pulse and blood examples were gathered inside three weeks before the commencement of 4-week intermittent fasting to survey the impact of not obligatory eating, toward the finish of fourth week during 4-week intermittent fasting to evaluate the impact of intermittent fasting and 1 after a long time following 4-week intermittent fasting to evaluate the vestige impact of intermittent fasting on serum proteome, parts of metabolic disorder, lipid and hepatic boards, and adiposity, oxidative pressure, and irritation biomarkers. At each time point, information on weight, abdomen circuit, and pulse and blood examples were gathered after in any event 8 h of fasting. The consistence with fasting was checked by a 13C-isotopic breath enhancement test, as recently depicted.

Proteomics in Serum

We recently depicted a vigorous, smoothed out proteomic way to deal with perform quantitative investigation of human serum tests utilizing Nano super elite fluid chromatography-couple mass spectrometry. Momentarily, 10 miniature liter of serum was hatched with the best 12 plentiful serum protein exhaustion unit and processed with trypsin on S-Trap segment. The processed peptide was eluted, vacuum dried, and fractionated utilizing high pH STAGE (Stop-and-go extraction) strategy into two pools, at that point exposed to Nano-HPLC–MS/MS investigation. The boundaries for mass spectrometry examination and the cycle for mass investigation is kept up equivalent to past distribution.

We likewise clarified the subtleties of the quality protein item (GP) measurement in our past distribution. Momentarily, we measured GPs utilizing the mark free, force based supreme evaluation (iBAQ) technique and afterward standardized to last quantificational esteem (FOT) characterized as the iBAQ worth of an individual protein isolated by the absolute iBAQ upsides of all distinguished proteins inside one investigation. The FOT addresses the overall wealth of every GP. The FOT upsides of a specific GP in various conditions (e.g., FOT worth of a GP before 4-week intermittent fasting and toward the finish of fourth week during 4-week intermittent fasting) can be separated to get a crease change. FOT esteem additionally gives the general evaluation of various GPs in a similar condition (e.g., FOT worth of two unique GPs toward the finish of fourth week during 4-week intermittent fasting).

Analysis of Stats

For factual examination of serum proteomics, we utilized Excel application. To decide genuinely altogether controlled protein levels toward the finish of fourth week during 4-week intermittent fasting and 1 after quite a while following 4-week intermittent fasting, we performed combined two-followed understudy's t-test utilizing log changed over iFOT esteems. We considered protein levels that showed an equivalent to or more prominent than fourfold normal matched change and a P esteem is critical. We played out a fountain of liquid magma plot investigation to show the GPs that had an equivalent to or more prominent than fourfold huge change toward the finish of 4-week intermittent fasting during 4-week intermittent fasting and 1 after a long time following 4-week intermittent fasting contrasted and the levels before 4-week intermittent fasting. Segments of metabolic disorder, lipid and hepatic boards, adiposity, oxidative pressure and irritation biomarkers

We estimated the parts of metabolic disorder, lipid board, hepatic board and adiposity, oxidative pressure, and aggravation biomarkers inside three weeks before 4-week intermittent fasting, toward the finish of 4-week intermittent fasting during 4-week intermittent fasting, and 1 after a long time following 4-week intermittent fasting. We assessed the insulin opposition by utilizing Homeostatic Model Assessment for Insulin Resistance (HOMA-IR) condition as portrayed by scientist. We determined the mean blood vessel pulse utilizing the accompanying equation.

We utilized SAS adaptation stage to perform factual examination of the parts of metabolic condition, lipid board, hepatic board, and adiposity, oxidative pressure, and aggravation biomarkers. We played out an understudy's combined t-test to decide measurably critical changes in the levels of the segments of metabolic disorder, lipid board, hepatic board, and adiposity, oxidative pressure, and irritation biomarkers estimated toward the finish of fourth week during 4-week intermittent fasting, and 1 after a long time following 4-week intermittent fasting. We determined Pearson's relationship coefficient to survey connections between huge GPs (i.e., GPs that showed critical overlap changes toward the finish of fourth week during 4-week intermittent fasting and 1 after quite a while following 4-week intermittent fasting) and the segments of metabolic disorder, lipid board, hepatic board, and adiposity, oxidative pressure, and irritation biomarkers. In these investigations, we considered a two-followed P worth of 0.05 measurably huge.

Subjects

We enlisted 14 subjects with metabolic disorder (8 guys: 6 females) with a mean age of 59 years. All subjects abstained for in excess of 14 h day by day for 29 days. Mean Fibro Scan CAP was 286 dB/m, and the mean versatile modulus was 9.7 kPa. Ten subjects had moderate to extreme hepatic steatosis, two had gentle hepatic steatosis (S1), and two had no hepatic steatosis (S0). F4 hepatic fibrosis was found in two subjects, F3 hepatic fibrosis in two, F2 hepatic fibrosis in one, and F0–F1 hepatic fibrosis in nine. Nine subjects were on enemy of hypertensive prescriptions; seven subjects were on subterranean insect diabetic meds, and six subjects were on statins.

Intermittent fasting from sunrise to nightfall (sunset) for about a month. Subjects abstained (no eating or drinking) for over 14 hours day by day for 29 days. The base required length of day by day fasting from first light to nightfall was 14 hours, 8 minutes for the briefest day, and 14 hours, 42 minutes for the longest day. Ramadan fasting is an interesting type of intermittent fasting from sunrise to (nightfall) without eating or drinking during the period of Ramadan dependent on the lunar schedule and has a few significant exceptional highlights: (1) Fasting is solely worked on during the human movement hours from sunrise to dusk and is for both eating and drinking, which separates the day break to dusk intermittent fasting from different types of intermittent fasting where eating quick bites and additionally drinking are permitted during the fasting window; (2) Although the principle suppers are at change time regions of the day (pre-sunrise breakfast and supper at dusk), eating and drinking outside these progress time regions is permitted as long all things considered inside the non-fasting window; (3) There is no interventional calorie or energy limitation; (4) Daily fasting window is in synchrony with circadian beat and earth's pivot on its hub on the grounds that the day by day quick beginnings at first light (the main change time region of the day) after a pre-sunrise breakfast and finishes at nightfall (sunset) (the subsequent progress time region of the day) with supper; (5) Monthly fasting window is in synchrony with the moon's turn around the earth and lunar stages on the grounds that the month to month fasting starts and closures when the new moon is located.

Normal Diet   Fasting Mimicking Diet Cycles

The base required span of every day fasting from sunrise to nightfall (sunset) was 14 hours, 8 minutes for the most limited day, and 14 hours, 42 minutes for the longest day. All subjects endured intermittent fasting great with no difficulties.

The Components of Oxidative stress, Lipids, Metabolic syndrome and Inflammation biomarkers

The mean levels of the parts of metabolic condition, lipid board, hepatic board, and adiposity, oxidative pressure, and irritation biomarkers before 4-week intermittent fasting and their mean combined changes toward the finish of fourth week during 4-week intermittent fasting and 1 after quite a while following 4-week intermittent fasting. There was a critical decrease in weight, weight list, abdomen boundary, systolic, diastolic and mean blood vessel blood pressures toward the finish of fourth week during 4-week intermittent fasting and a huge decrease in weight, weight file, midriff periphery and HOMA-IR, 1 after quite a while following 4-week intermittent fasting contrasted and the levels before 4-week intermittent fasting. We noticed a decrease in insulin, glucose, HOMA-IR, fatty oil, leptin, and a few oxidative pressure and irritation biomarker levels and an increment in high-thickness lipoprotein and adiponectin levels toward the finish of fourth week during 4-week intermittent fasting, be that as it may, these boundaries didn't arrive at factual importance.

Serum Protein Study

The proteome inclusion and its dynamic request of normal iFOT esteems from the examples taken toward the finish of fourth week during 4-week intermittent fasting. There were 1219 GPs recuperated with more than eight significant degrees of dynamic reach. There was a huge normal combined crease change in the levels of a few GPs toward the finish of fourth week during 4-week intermittent fasting contrasted and the levels before 4-week intermittent fasting. The chose ones from these GPs related with tumor concealment, carcinogenesis, DNA fix, and insulin flagging. GP levels toward the finish of fourth week during 4-week intermittent fasting contrasted and the levels before 4-week intermittent fasting. We discovered huge decline in DNA polymerase, antimicrobial peptide and nucleolar protein interfacing GP levels contrasted and the levels before 4-week intermittent fasting.

Quality protein items (GP) recuperated toward the finish of fourth week during 4-week intermittent fasting and one after a long time following 4-week intermittent fasting. (A) Distribution of standardized relative GP sum and area of zeroed in altogether expanded or diminished proteins in serum tests taken toward the finish of fourth week during 4-week intermittent fasting GP name and rank order are shown.

(B) Volcano plot shows chosen GPs that had an equivalent to or more prominent than fourfold critical change (blue and red tones address a huge abatement and expansion in the degrees of GPs, separately) toward the finish of fourth week during 4-week intermittent fasting contrasted and the levels before 4-week intermittent fasting. (C) Distribution of standardized relative GP sum and area of zeroed in fundamentally expanded or diminished proteins in serum tests required 1 after a long time following 4-week intermittent fasting appeared in GP name and rank request. (D) Volcano plot shows chosen GPs that had an equivalent to or more noteworthy than fourfold huge change (blue and red tones address a critical decline and expansion in the degrees of GPs, individually) 1 after quite a while following 4-week intermittent fasting contrasted and the levels before 4-week intermittent fasting.

The proteome inclusion and its dynamic request from 14 examples gathered 1 after a long time following 4-week intermittent fasting. There were 1216 GPs recuperated with more than eight significant degrees of dynamic reach. There was a critical normal combined crease change in the levels of a few GPs 1 after quite a while following 4-week intermittent fasting contrasted and the levels before 4-week intermittent fasting. It is shown chosen ones from these GPs related with tumor concealment, carcinogenesis, and insulin flagging, and delayed life expectancy.

There was a huge normal matched overlay change in the levels of a few GPs 1 after quite a while following 4-week intermittent fasting contrasted and the levels toward the finish of fourth week during 4-week intermittent fasting. It showed the normal combined overlay changes in the chose GPs 1 after a long time following 4-week intermittent fasting contrasted and the levels toward the finish of fourth week during 4-week intermittent fasting.

Correlations between GPs and Oxidative stress, Lipids, Metabolic syndrome and Inflammation biomarkers

A few GPs that showed critical normal combined overlap changes toward the finish of fourth week during 4-week intermittent fasting and 1 after quite a while following 4-week intermittent fasting were associated with the segments of metabolic disorder, lipid and hepatic boards and adiposity, oxidative pressure and irritation biomarkers toward the finish of fourth week during 4-week intermittent fasting and 1 after quite a while following 4-week intermittent fasting. There was no critical connection between log 2 overlay changes in the chose proteins and changes in weight, abdomen periphery and weight file toward the finish of fourth week during 4-week intermittent fasting and 1 after a long time following 4-week intermittent fasting contrasted and pattern.

1.4 Intermittent Fasting and Anticancer Serum Proteomic Signature

We announced the consequences of the principal human investigation of serum proteomics of 4-week intermittent fasting from sunrise to nightfall led in subjects with metabolic disorder. The outcomes showed that intermittent fasting from first light to dusk for in excess of 14 h every day for four sequential weeks instigated a one of a kind anticancer, hostile to diabetes and against maturing proteomic reaction, up managed a few administrative proteins that assume a critical part in tumor concealment, DNA fix, humoral guard, insulin flagging, and down directed a few tumor advertiser proteins. These progressions in protein articulation are likely identified with the rest of the circadian clock beat by intermittent fasting from sunrise to dusk and in accordance with the consequences of past murine examinations.

Discussion

This pilot study has significant clinical ramifications, explicitly from the point of view of kind of intermittent fasting on malignancy avoidance in subjects with metabolic condition. There are two significant types of day by day intermittent fasting dependent on an opportunity to begin and end fasting: (1) Fasting that begins at sunrise and closures at nightfall (sunset).

The fasting window is between two even change time regions of the day (first light and nightfall) which is the human action time frame; (2) Fasting that begins at a self-decided time and goes on for a fixed number of hours comprising of both human movement (daytime) and inertia (evening time) periods (e.g., 16:8 intermittent fasting that begins at 8 pm and closures around early afternoon).

Ramadan fasting is a novel type of intermittent fasting from sunrise to nightfall (sunset) without eating or drinking during the period of Ramadan dependent on the lunar schedule and has a few significant one of a kind highlights: (1) Fasting is only worked on during the human action hours from first light to dusk (sunset) and is for both eating and drinking, which separates the sunrise to dusk intermittent fasting from different types of intermittent fasting where drinking as well as eating quick bites are permitted during the fasting window; (2) Although the principle suppers are at the progress time regions of the day (pre-first light breakfast and supper at nightfall), eating (e.g., bites) and drinking outside these change time regions is permitted as long all things considered inside the non-fasting window; (3) There is no interventional calorie or energy limitation; (4) Daily fasting window is in synchrony with circadian cadence and earth's pivot on its hub on the grounds that the everyday quick beginnings at first light (the main progress time region of the day) after a pre-sunrise breakfast and finishes at dusk (sunset) (the subsequent change time region of the day) with supper; (5) Monthly fasting window is in synchrony with the moon's turn around the earth and lunar stages in light of the fact that the month to month fasting starts and closures when the new moon is located. It is gathered that this fasting design brings about energy holds being gotten to without prompting micronutrient insufficiencies because of renewal after nightfall.

Fasting during action hours of the day has all the earmarks of being of fundamental significance in malignancy anticipation and treatment. An investigation showed that subject with no admittance to food during the movement period of a 12 hours light/12-h dull cycle had a fundamentally slower tumor movement and higher endurance contrasted and subject that had no admittance to food during the latency stage, and subject that approached food not obligatory. The most noteworthy anticancer reaction happened in the subject with no admittance to food during the action stage, and the more awful result was in the subject that approached food not indispensable. There was a minor anticancer impact and no endurance advantage in the subject with no admittance to food during the inertia stage. Concerning people, an investigation led among 2413 ladies with bosom disease without diabetes mellitus showed that fasting equivalent to or more than 13 hours around evening time (the mix of dormancy and action hours) was related with a decreased danger of bosom malignant growth repeat. Of note, this examination didn't have control subjects who abstained only during the action hours (daytime). Out and out, these creature and human investigations show that intermittent fasting either during day by day movement or idleness hours (with or without reaching out to action hours) have an anticancer impact contrasted and not indispensable eating; nonetheless, the most vigorous anticancer reaction seems to happen when delayed fasting is polished only during the action hours.

As per the discoveries of these murine and human investigations, we tracked down a huge overlay expansion in the degrees of explicit tumor silencer/anticancer proteins toward the finish of fourth week during 4-week intermittent fasting from day break to dusk as well as 1 after a long time following 4-week intermittent fasting from first light to nightfall, that are down managed in a few diseases bringing about malignant growth metastasis and helpless guess. The CALR quality encodes for calreticulin, which is a calcium-restricting protein situated in the endoplasmic reticulum and core. Malignancy cells labeled by calreticulin on their surface animate an immunogenic disease cell demise by empowering their phagocytosis by the dendritic cells of the safe framework which thus triggers T-cell-interceded safe reaction. It is showed that anthracyclines move calreticulin to the tumor cell surface, and trigger immunogenic tumor cell demise ("eat me" signal).

CALU quality encodes for calumenin, a calcium-restricting protein that assumes a critical part in the endoplasmic reticulum capacities, including collapsing and arranging of proteins. Calumenin is an inhibitor of cell relocation and metastasis in a few malignancies, e.g., hepatocellular, pancreatic, head and neck squamous cell, and lung squamous cell carcinomas. INTS6 quality encodes for a DEAD box RNA helicase. It is a tumor silencer quality that plays a huge tumor-suppressive job in hepatocellular carcinoma and prostate malignancy. The acceptance of INTS6 quality was appeared to smother maiming safe prostate disease. Changes in KIT are connected to a few diseases, and the deficiency of proto-oncogene c-KIT articulation has been related with helpless anticipation in bosom malignant growth.

A few other anticancer GPs require elaboration. CROCC is a tumor-silencer quality that was appeared to smother hepatocellular carcinoma by means of pathway enactment. The down guideline of CROCC was related with helpless endurance in patients with hepatocellular carcinoma after careful resection. PIGR that encodes for polymeric immunoglobulin receptor was discovered to be down controlled in pancreatic and periampullary adenocarcinoma and cellular breakdown in the lungs. The up guideline of IGFBP4 (encodes for a protein that ties insulin-like development factors), was appeared to work as a powerful tumor silencer in hepatocellular carcinoma and postpone tumor arrangement in prostate malignant growth cells. SEMA4B is engaged with protein-coding and encodes for a protein that represses tumor development in non-little cell cellular breakdown in the lungs.

A huge overlay decrease in the levels of a few tumor advertiser/favorable to malignant growth GPs was seen toward the finish of fourth week during 4-week intermittent fasting and additionally multi week after fulfillment of 4-week intermittent fasting. These incorporate that are up controlled in a few diseases bringing about metastasis and helpless anticipation.

POLK quality encodes for a specific DNA polymerase. Particular DNA polymerases are ectopically overexpressed in a few diseases, can work as an oncogene and upgrade changes initiated by DNA harm. Overexpression of POLK has been accounted for in cellular breakdown in the lungs. POLK overexpression adds to malignancy advancement by inactivating wild-type p53, and this was appeared in cellular breakdown in the lungs. POLK quality additionally assumes a part in bosom malignant growth. A case–control study showed a higher danger of creating bosom malignant growth in ladies with two explicit single nucleotide polymorphisms in the POLK quality contrasted and controls. NIFK that encodes for a protein that capacities in mitosis and movement of cell cycle was discovered to be up controlled and connected with helpless anticipation in cellular breakdown in the lungs. SRGN encodes for a proteoglycan in hematopoietic cells and its overexpression is related with helpless anticipation in hepatocellular, colorectal malignancy, non-little cell cellular breakdown in the lungs, and nasopharyngeal carcinoma. CAMP that is otherwise called LL37 and

CAP18, encodes for cathelicidin antimicrobial peptide. CAMP was appeared to expand the development of colon malignancy by means of catenin flagging pathway enactment and capacity as a tumor advertiser for lung and ovarian diseases. CD109 encodes for a glycosyl phosphatidylinositol-connected glycoprotein that was discovered to be overexpressed in a few tumors, e.g., dangerous melanoma, squamous cell carcinoma of the lung and oral cavity. PLAC1, which has a one-sided articulation in placenta, was demonstrated to be communicated in hepatocellular carcinoma, and overexpressed in bosom disease, non-little cell cellular breakdown in the lungs, and pancreatic ductal adenocarcinoma.

Intermittent Fasting Role in Humoral Defense against (SARS-CoV)

Calreticulin was appeared to upgrade IgG-interceded invulnerable reaction when it is intertwined with spike (S) protein of SARS-CoV64. Recombinant combination protein that joins calreticulin and SARS-CoV S protein 450–650 section had a lot higher immunogenicity when contrasted and SARS-CoV S protein alone64. We tracked down a normal 16-crease expansion in the CALR GP level multi week after culmination of 4-week intermittent fasting contrasted and the level before 4-week intermittent fasting. Our discoveries, joined with the earlier report, recommend that 4-week IF can assume a significant part in humoral protection against SARS-CoV, and further examinations are required.

Intermittent Fasting induces Insulin Signaling and Improves Insulin Resistance

Four-week intermittent fasting incited key administrative proteins of insulin flagging, including VPS8, POLRMT and IGFBP5 toward the finish of fourth week during 4-week intermittent fasting and PRKCSH 1 after quite a while following 4-week intermittent fasting. The enlistment of VPS8, POLRMT, and IGFBP5 GPs toward the finish of fourth week during 4-week intermittent fasting went before the critical decrease in insulin opposition assessed by HOMA-IR that happened 1 after quite a while following 4-week intermittent fasting. VPS8, a subunit of CORVET complex, assumes a basic part in integrin requiring cell attachment and movement, and reusing of beta-1 integrin. Integrin are transmembrane receptors interfacing the extracellular framework to the actin cytoskeleton of the cells and in this way going about as a sensor for cell grip. An impeded integrin motioning in the extracellular grid of skeletal muscle, fat tissue and liver can prompt insulin opposition. An unblemished skeletal muscle and beta-cell mitochondrial work is imperative for insulin amalgamation. Type 2 diabetes mellitus is related with skeletal muscle mitochondrial brokenness and diminished oxidative limit. POLRMT encodes for the mitochondrial RNA polymerase that assumes a basic part in record in pancreatic beta-cells and insulin emission in the pancreas. As the deficiency of POLRMT results in serious mitochondrial brokenness in heart muscle, a comparable mitochondrial brokenness ought to happen in beta-cells with the misfortune or brokenness of POLRMT, bringing about insulin obstruction and diabetes mellitus. IGFBP5 assumes a functioning part in myoblast separation by restricting to insulin development factor II and up directing its demeanor. PRKCSH encodes for a protein called hepatocystin or 80K-H, which is a beta subunit of glucosidase and substrate for protein kinase C26, that assumes a vital part in GLUT4 vesicle dealing (movement of GLUT4 to the plasma film) in the insulin flagging pathway 72 by framing a complex with 80K-H Overexpression of the hepatocystin 1 after quite a while following 4-week intermittent fasting is reminiscent of progress of insulin motioning through improvement of GLUT4 vesicle dealing. The up guideline of PRKCSH GPs corresponded with the improvement in HOMA-IR 1 after quite a while following 4-week intermittent fasting.

Intermittent Fasting with Autophagy and Oxidative Stress Parameters

Autophagy gives off an impression of being one of the instruments of intermittent fasting in malignancy avoidance. Down guideline of the hepatocystin encoded by PRKCSH results in useless glucosidase II, and along these lines expansion in autophagy through subordinate pathway. The way that we discovered decrease toward the finish of fourth week during 4-week intermittent fasting and afterward 73-crease expansion in PRKCSH GP level 1 after quite a while following 4-week intermittent fasting is reminiscent of expanded autophagy during 4-week intermittent fasting and diminished autophagy with the subjects' re-visitation of not obligatory eating. In spite of the fact that it didn't arrive at measurable importance, we discovered a decrease in numerous oxidative pressure and irritation biomarkers just as gamma-glutamyl transferase levels, recommending glutathione repletion toward the finish of fourth week during 4-week intermittent fasting.

Intermittent fasting regulates proteins associated with prolonged longevity and DNA repair

We noticed a normal six overlay expansion in H2B histone GP levels 1 after quite a while following 4-week intermittent fasting contrasted and the levels before 4-week intermittent fasting. It is exhibited comparable discoveries in yeast cells. They detailed that histone proteins are lost in maturing yeast cells, while histone protein overexpression and providing additional histone proteins delayed life span. Creators proposed that additional histone protein supply expands life expectancy by giving a tighter chromatin bundling, and in this manner reestablishing the transcriptional hushing that is lost in maturing. We additionally noticed a critical positive relationship between H2B histone GP levels and high-thickness lipoprotein levels 1 after a long time following 4-week intermittent fasting. The relationship between high-thickness lipoprotein levels and life span was recently revealed. Our discoveries of a critical positive relationship between H2B histone GP and high-thickness lipoprotein levels 1 after a long time following 4-week intermittent fasting shed light on the unthinking comprehension of the relationship between high-thickness lipoprotein levels and life span. Other than the all-inclusive life expectancy, the overexpression of histone proteins may likewise be related with expanded DNA articulation and fix since light prompted DNA harm was appeared to down direct histone quality record through the G1 designated spot pathway. Also, we noticed a normal 74-crease expansion in the AP5Z1 GP level toward the finish of fourth week during 4-week intermittent fasting contrasted and the level before 4-week intermittent fasting. AP5Z1 is a helicase that probably assumes a part in the maintenance of homologous recombination DNA twofold strand break. A variation in the AP5Z1 quality was related with outrageous life span in a genome-wide affiliation study led among 75,000 members of the UK bio bank.

1.5 Limitations and Strength

The qualities of our examination are as per the following: (1) we played out a strong, smoothed out proteomics strategy to evaluate proteins in the human serum utilizing Nano UHPLC-MS/MS15. With this one of a kind proteomics strategy, we had the option to recuperate in excess of 1000 GPs toward the finish of the fourth week during 4-week intermittent fasting and 1 after quite a while following 4-week intermittent fasting; (2) We assessed serum proteome at the same time with the parts of metabolic condition, lipid, and hepatic boards, and adiposity, oxidative pressure, and irritation biomarkers; (3) We evaluated the vestige impact of 4-week intermittent fasting in the wake of changing to not obligatory eating. For this, we thought about the GP levels estimated 1 after a long time following 4-week intermittent fasting with the levels estimated toward the finish of fourth week during 4-week intermittent fasting. A few GPs that had a critical overlay change toward the finish of fourth week during 4-week intermittent fasting contracted and the levels before 1 week intermittent fasting, didn't have any huge crease change 1 after a long time following 4-week intermittent fasting contrasted and the levels toward the finish of fourth week during 4-week intermittent fasting (e.g., CALU, CAMP). These discoveries recommend that intermittent fasting has a remainder impact on these proteins. Then again, a few GPs that had no huge crease change toward the finish of fourth week during 4-week intermittent fasting contrasted and the levels before 4-week intermittent fasting, had a critical overlap change 1 after quite a while following 4-week intermittent fasting contrasted and the levels toward the finish of fourth week during 4-week intermittent fasting (e.g., PRKCSH, HIST1H2BA). These discoveries may propose either diminished or deferred remainder impact of intermittent fasting on the proteome. There is likewise a likelihood that intermittent fasting may have set off a course of proteomic changes in a continuum that may not be clarified by the evaluation of the serum proteome at a solitary time point alone after intermittent fasting is halted.

A few GPs that showed huge overlay changes in subjects with metabolic condition had likewise shown comparative changes (e.g., increment or diminishing) toward the finish of fourth week during 30-day intermittent fasting and multi week following 30-day intermittent fasting in our past investigation led in sound subjects in spite of the fact that they had not arrived at measurable importance.

The absence of caloric estimation by dietary appraisal is one of the impediments of our examination. The improvement in the segments of metabolic condition could incompletely be clarified by the huge weight decrease. In any case, we didn't track down any critical relationship between log 2 crease changes in the chose proteins and changes in weight, midriff circuit and weight record toward the finish of fourth week during 4-week intermittent fasting and 1 after quite a while following 4-week intermittent fasting contrasted and gauge recommending that the impact of 4-week intermittent fasting from sunrise to dusk on the proteomic changes was autonomous of weight decrease. Moreover, our past investigation led in sound volunteers who abstained from first light to nightfall for 30 days showed the acceptance of an anticancer proteome without a huge weight change. We assessed insulin opposition by HOMA-IR condition as opposed to playing out an oral glucose resistance test. A non-critical decrease in HOMA-IR toward the finish of fourth week during 4-week intermittent fasting may be identified with inadequate precision of the HOMA-IR condition in our examination populace. HOMA-IR condition was found to have restricted exactness in grown-ups between the ages 60 and 88 and subjects on insulin treatment (except if the glucose and insulin are in consistent state levels in subjects on insulin). Given the way that 11 out of 14 examination subjects were 60 years of age or more established and one subject was on insulin treatment, HOMA-IR may have belittled the decrease in insulin obstruction that happened toward the finish of fourth week during 4-week intermittent fasting.

Regardless, there was a decrease in glucose, insulin, and HOMA-IR levels toward the finish of fourth week during 4-week intermittent fasting. Albeit these discoveries didn't arrive at factual importance, they give extra proof to the insect diabetic impact of the 4-week intermittent fasting from day break to dusk.

1.6 Intermittent Fasting Enhance Immunotherapy

There is developing interest in outfitting way of life and drug intercessions to support resistant capacity, lessen tumor development, and improve malignant growth treatment adequacy while diminishing treatment poisonousness. Mediations focusing on glucose digestion are especially encouraging, as they can possibly straightforwardly restrain tumor cell multiplication. In any case, since hostile to tumor insusceptible effector cells additionally depend on glycolysis to support their clonal extension and capacity, it stays indistinct whether glucose-regulating treatments will uphold or thwart against tumor invulnerability. In this point of view, we sum up a developing assortment of writing that assesses the impacts of intermittent fasting, calorie limitation mimetic, and against hyperglycemic specialists on enemy of tumor invulnerability and immunotherapy results. In light of the restricted information at present accessible, we fight that extra pre-clinical examinations and clinical preliminaries are justified to address the impacts of co organization of against hyperglycemic specialists or glucose-bringing down way of life changes on enemy of tumor resistance and disease treatment results. We stress that there is presently deficient proof to give proposals with respect to these mediations to malignant growth patients going through immunotherapy. Notwithstanding, whenever discovered to be protected and viable in clinical preliminaries, intercessions focusing on glucose digestion could go about as minimal effort combinatorial adjuvants for malignancy patients accepting resistant designated spot barricade or different immunotherapies.

Malignancy envelops an expansive group of illnesses that include strange and unregulated cell multiplication. Scientists have point by point the basic qualities that all diseases have, including supported proliferative signs, dysregulated cell energetics, and aversion of invulnerable interceded slaughtering, tumor-advancing aggravation, intrusion, and metastasis. These components advance a feed-forward circle preferring an invulnerable dodging microenvironment that upholds tumor movement. The harmony between defensive enemy of tumor systems and tumor-advancing/immunosuppressive variables is basic for directing disease movement or abatement.

CR is normally characterized as a decrease in every day energy admission of at any rate 10–20% underneath standard not indispensable taking care of, without inciting hunger. CR has been investigated in pre-clinical and clinical examinations for its capacity to broaden life expectancy and improve cardio metabolic wellbeing and is currently being investigated for its enemy of malignancy properties.

1.7 Intermittent Fasting target Glucose Metabolism to Improve Immunotherapies

Disease immunotherapies are intended to improve the defensive resistant reactions that can kill set up tumors and are promising therapy alternatives for some malignant growths. Malignancy immunotherapy contains various methodologies, including cytokine treatments, directed antibodies, supportive cell moves, hereditarily designed fanciful antigen receptor (CAR) T cells, disease immunizations, hereditarily designed oncolytic infections, and invulnerable designated spot barricade (ICB). Victories have been seen inside every class; be that as it may, ICB-based treatments are the most often used immunotherapy and are as of now FDA-affirmed as therapy choices in patients with numerous sorts of cutting edge diseases. ICB utilizes antibodies to upset the receptor/ligand matches that convey inhibitory messages to effector T cells (e.g., Programmed Death-1 [PD-1] and Programmed Death-Ligand 1 [PD-L1]). Regardless of exhibited clinical advantage, normally half of patients accepting ICB experience unbiased, sturdy reactions. This test has prompted a significant push to improve ICB adequacy by creating novel combinatorial therapy procedures to decrease disease cell practicality and multiplication, increment tumor invasion by effector T cells, as well as advance T cell effector work in the tumor microenvironment.

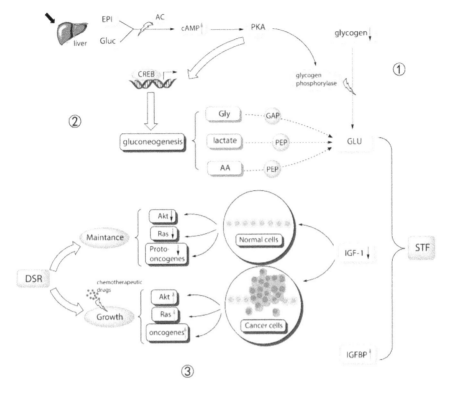

One combinatorial methodology that has gathered a lot of consideration lately is the utilization of glucose-restricting way of life changes or against diabetic medications (summed up in Table 1) that can be co-controlled with immunotherapy. The reasoning fundamental this methodology is that tumor cells are frequently subject to glucose as an essential fuel source. This glycolytic reliance emerges from the consistent multiplication of tumor cells, which requires continuous admittance to energy and the structure squares of cell biomass. To meet these prerequisites, disease cells use glycolysis, even within the sight of oxygen, a cycle alluded to as vigorous glycolysis or the "Warburg impact". Accordingly, way of life and pharmacologic intercessions that diminish intra-tumoral glucose levels may moderate malignant growth cell replication and render disease cells more defenseless to insusceptible intervened slaughtering, along these lines boosting the viability of immunotherapy.

A significant worry with any treatment approach zeroed in on restricting glucose accessibility is that it might have accidental adverse results for defensive invulnerability. This is on the grounds that effector CD8+ T cells additionally depend on glucose-subordinate, Warburg-style digestion for their clonal extension and hostile to malignancy capacities, including cytolytic action and cytokine discharge. Earlier examinations report that dysregulated CD8+ T cell digestion inside the tumor microenvironment impedes T cell effector works and advances tumor movement. For example, in treatment-innocent human subjects with clear cell renal cell carcinoma, tumor-invading CD8+ T cells show a deficiency of proliferative limit because of metabolic deformities, including debilitated glucose take-up and glycolytic limit; divided and hyperpolarized mitochondria; and expanded creation of responsive oxygen species. These perceptions loan legitimacy to worries that further limits of intra-tumoral glucose will hinder both T cell and tumor cell digestion. Nonetheless, an exquisite investigation by Chang et al. given proof that ICB may specifically shield T cells from diminished glucose accessibility inside the tumor microenvironment.

In this report, the creators represented that ICB organization with either hostile to CTLA-4, against PD-1, or hostile to PD-L1 improved the glycolytic limit and Interferon-gamma (IFN) creation of CD8+ tumor-invading T cells. A similar report discovered that enemy of PD-L1 restrained glucose take-up and glycolysis in tumor cells. Along these lines, ICB may differentially modify the metabolic programming of tumor cells versus hostile to tumor resistant cells to support malignancy relapse. This perception makes ICB an especially alluring sort of immunotherapy to consolidate with glucose-restricting way of life mediations or against diabetic medications, as the outcome might be debilitated tumor cell digestion and suitability, with associatively improved T cell digestion and effector work.

Notwithstanding, it stays muddled whether intercessions that lower plasma glucose apply a net positive or adverse consequence on tumor multiplication, hostile to tumor resistance, and malignant growth immunotherapy results, especially with regards to ICB. Insignificant pre-clinical information exists, and no clinical preliminaries have been directed to decide whether glucose-restricting way of life intercessions or hostile to diabetic medications collaborate with other immunotherapy stages, as receptive cell treatments, malignancy immunizations, or CAR T cells. These immunotherapy methodologies may drive an immunometabolic profile more vulnerable to decreases in glucose accessibility; thusly, expansive clearing ends can't be drawn on the pertinence and security of glucose-focusing on treatments as an adjuvant to all immunotherapy techniques. Underneath, we survey pre-clinical information in regards with the impacts of glucose-bringing down intercessions on tumor cell expansion and against tumor resistance. A few reports have demonstrated that glucose-administrative intercessions may really improve the adequacy of ICB and perhaps different sorts of immunotherapy. When accessible, we additionally give data about human subject information or continuous clinical preliminaries that are exploring these mediations in malignant growth patients. Considering the developing utilization of hostile to hyperglycemic specialists and flooding well known interest in intermittent fasting and calorie limitation mimetics, we center our conversation around this subset of promising mediations. Albeit other focused on treatments, similar to tyrosine kinase inhibitors (e.g.,

PI3K inhibitors), are promising for balancing flagging falls pertinent to glucose digestion and for affecting resistant reactions following immunotherapy, these intercessions were not talked about here in light of the fact that their essential methods of activity are not glucose guideline.

1.8 Pre and Post Clinical Findings

Bountiful proof from creature models exhibits that CR lessens malignancy occurrence and postpones disease movement through different instruments. For instance, CR can hinder malignancy cell multiplication by diminishing plasma glucose and insulin, which thus adjusts articulation of cell cycle proteins, alters tumor silencer quality capacity, and disturbs metabolic pathways. CR can likewise decrease insulin-like development factor-1 (IGF-1), a supplement detecting development factor that is invigorated by glucose. IGF-1 actuates flagging pathways in carcinogenic cells to advance glycolysis and tumor cell multiplication, while at the same time hindering apoptosis. Subsequently, the pleiotropic impacts of CR combine to dull the proliferative limit of tumor cells. Pre-clinical information recommend that CR can sharpen carcinogenic cells to radiotherapy and chemotherapy by adversely directing enemy of apoptotic protection instruments. Furthermore, it is accounted for that persistent CR protected antigen-explicit CD4 T cell preparing and prompted a huge endurance advantage when joined with hostile to OX40 (CD134) immunotherapy in matured tumor-bearing subject. Thusly, CR appears to both restrain tumor cell multiplication and keep up enemy of tumor resistance and can possibly be joined with immunotherapy dependent on this pre-clinical finding.

Regardless of the possibility to upgrade immunotherapies, worries about loss of lean mass and antipathy for CR limit helpful interpretation to malignancy patients who may as of now be battling with cachexia and loss of craving. Gainful impacts have been seen in an adjuvant setting when joined with focused treatment or chemotherapy; notwithstanding, until this point in time, there have been no preliminaries analyzing the impacts of CR on ICB in people. Subsequently, it isn't evident whether CR can be securely joined with ICB or different immunotherapies to improve patient results. Given the opportunities for CR to speed up cachexia in disease patients, such investigations ought to be drawn closer with alert.

Chapter 2. Mechanism and Role of Intermittent Fasting in Tumors

Intermittent fasting (IF) is turning into a common subject around the world, as it can cause changes in the body's energy digestion measures, improve wellbeing, and influence the movement of numerous illnesses, especially in the condition of oncology. Late examination has shown that IF can adjust the energy digestion of tumor cells, in this way hindering tumor development and improving antitumor resistant reactions. Besides, IF can build malignant growth affectability to chemotherapy and radiotherapy and diminish the results of these customary anticancer therapies. On the off chance that is thusly arising as a promising way to deal with clinical disease treatment. Nonetheless, the harmony between long haul advantages of IF contrasted and the damage from deficient caloric admission isn't surely known. In this article, we audit the job of IF in tumorigenesis and tumor treatment, and examine some logical issues that stay to be explained, which may give some help with the use of IF in clinical tumor treatment.

2.1 Introduction

Intermittent fasting (IF) is an eating regimen based treatment that switches back and forth among fasting and free taking care of/eating for a while. This training was created by individuals looking for pragmatic and moderately safe fasting strategies to accomplish day by day caloric limitation. On the off chance that regimens for the most part incorporate transient intermittent fasting [such as 16–18 h of day by day fasting, substitute day fasting or 5:2 IF (2 days a week)], long haul intermittent fasting, etc. Over a century prior, Moreschi previously portrayed the useful impacts of fasting and confining caloric admission on tumors in creatures. In 1997, found that diminishing food accessibility over a long period (caloric limitation, CR) effectsly affected maturing and the life expectancy of creatures. Follow-up examinations have therefore showed that IF over a time of 12 h to half a month can forestall sicknesses and defer maturing in numerous organic entities (like microorganisms, yeasts, worms, and subject). In particular, intermittent fasting IF can improve the capacity of the whole body, including tissues and organs. Additionally, in the wake of directing an IF routine, a few tissues and organs are more impervious to an assortment of hurtful upgrades that include metabolic, oxidative, ionic, awful, and proteotoxic stresses. Creature model investigations of test sicknesses have additionally shown that intermittent fasting IF can ease the advancement of numerous ongoing illnesses, including heftiness, diabetes, vascular infections, malignancy, and neurodegenerative sicknesses.

From an unthinking viewpoint, considers have exhibited that the impact of IF is identified with the versatile energy metabolic reaction of organs, tissues, and cells set off by intermittent fasting IF (basically the metabolic change from glucose to ketone bodies as a fuel source), which shows as expanded ketone body creation, autophagy, DNA fix, and hostile to push capacities, and cancer prevention agent protection is upgraded in the beginning phase of IF. During times of recuperation (counting eating and resting), the change from ketones to glucose as the primary fuel wellspring of cells brings about an improved capacity to deliver glucose and incorporate intracellular proteins and expanded articulation and mitochondrial biogenesis. During the drawn out variation time frame, the insulin affectability of cells and body protection from insulin are expanded, blood glucose homeostasis and lipid digestion are additionally improved, and stomach fat and irritation are decreased. These cycles are joined by modifications in the insulin-like development factor-1 flagging pathway, a decline in leptin levels, an expansion in adiponectin levels, an improvement in enemy of stress capacity, an abatement in free extreme creation, development and utilitarian rebuilding, and an increment in body protection from stress.

The impact of various times of intermittent fasting (IF). In the beginning phase of IF, the impact of IF primarily happens through ketogenesis, which shows as expanded ketone body creation, autophagy, and DNA fix, just as upgraded against pressure capacities and cancer prevention agent protection. During times of recuperation (counting eating and resting), the fundamental fuel wellsprings of cells are changed over from ketones to glucose, which prompts expanded glucose, articulation, and mitochondrial biogenesis, upgraded capacity to incorporate intracellular proteins, and rebuilt development and capacities. During the drawn out variation time frame, the insulin affectability of cells and body protection from stress are expanded, blood glucose homeostasis and lipid digestion are additionally improved, and stomach fat and aggravation are diminished.

A new report announced that the miRNA hardware, especially the miRNA-handling catalyst drsh-1, is associated with fasting-actuated changes in quality articulation and IF-prompted life span. This investigation found that miRISC parts and the miRNA-handling protein, drsh-1, are up managed by fasting, proposing that the miRNA apparatus is initiated because of fasting. The outflow of miRNA hardware proteins in mouse fat tissues has been accounted for to diminish with maturing, and these abatements are smothered by CR. Additionally, miRNA cluster investigations uncovered that the articulation levels of various miRNAs changed following 2 days of fasting. These outcomes show that segments of the miRNA hardware, particularly the miRNA-preparing protein, drsh-1, and miRNA particles, may assume significant parts in intervening IF-actuated life span through the guideline of fasting-incited changes in quality articulation.

2.2 Intermittent Fasting and Growth of Tumor

Late investigations have shown that intermittent fasting IF can influence the energy digestion of tumor cells and restrain tumor cell development, and can likewise improve the capacity of insusceptible cells and advance antitumor resistant reactions, which demonstrates that IF has possible worth in tumor immunotherapy.

The atomic system by which IF represses tumor cell development is as per the following. CR actuated by IF represses the IGF-1/AKT and mTORC1 pathways in tumor cells, while (AMP) enacted protein kinase (AMPK), which is subject to the nicotinamide adenine dinucleotide coenzyme deacetylase-1 (Sirtuin-1, SIRT1) and SIRT3 pathways, is initiated, subsequently ruining tumor cell development. Remarkably, AMPK and SIRTs rely upon one another in IF-related metabolic variation. AMPK can prompt actuation of SIRT1 through (NAMPT), while SIRT1 can initiate AMPK through liver kinase B1 (LKB1) guideline. Furthermore, FOXO3a (a downstream particle of SIRT1 and SIRT3) and AMPK can each improve the other's transcriptional activities36. SIRT3 represses tumor development by enacting FOXO3a and the statement of superoxide dismutase 2 (SOD2), along these lines lessening the degree of responsive oxygen species (ROS) and contrarily controlling the outflow of hypoxia inducible factor-1 (HIF-1). SIRT3 enacts SOD2 by means of up guideline of FOXO3a. Moreover, IF can specifically restrain tumor development by up controlling leptin receptor (LEPR) and its downstream flagging pathway protein, PR/SET area quality family 1 (PRDM1).

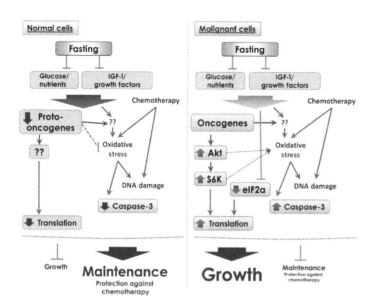

The sub-atomic component by which intermittent fasting (IF) influences tumor cell development. Unthinkingly, IF restrains the IGF-1/AKT and mTORC1 pathways in tumor cells, while the AMPK, SIRT1, and SIRT3 pathways are enacted. Likewise, AMPK and SIRTs rely upon one another in IF-related metabolic transformation. In any case, AMPK can actuate enactment of SIRT1 through NAMPT, while SIRT1 can initiate AMPK through LKB1 guideline. FOXO3a (a downstream particle of SIRT1 and SIRT3) and AMPK can each upgrade the other's transcriptional exercises. Besides, SIRT3 represses tumor development by enacting FOXO3a and the statement of superoxide dismutase (SOD), subsequently decreasing the degree of receptive oxygen species and adversely controlling the declaration of HIF-1. SIRT3 initiates SOD2 by means of up guideline of FOXO3a. Besides, IF can specifically hinder tumor development by up managing LEPR and its downstream flagging pathway protein, PRDM1.

In any case, the significant declines in glucose, insulin, and IGF-1 brought about by fasting, which is joined by cell passing as well as decay in a wide scope of tissues and organs, including the liver and kidneys, is trailed by a time of strangely high cell multiplication in these tissues, driven to a limited extent by the renewal of development factors during re-taking care of. When joined with cancer-causing agents during re-taking care of, this expanded proliferative action can increment carcinogenesis as well as precancerous sores in tissues, including the liver and colon. What's more, some past investigations have shown that intermittent fasting IF neglects to restrain the arrangement of carcinomas in subject. Along with these investigations, we subsequently theorize that over the top utilization of IF may have the contrary impact in restraining the event of tumors. To sum up, it is recommended that the system by which IF represses tumor development is intricate, and the particular atomic components that add to explicit tumors might be distinctive when unique IF or CR regimens are carried out.

2.3 Intermittent Fasting and Immunity of Tumor

Resistant departure is a vital factor in tumorigenesis. Studies have shown that intermittent fasting IF can influence the turn of events and capacity of an assortment of resistant cells, in this manner directing antitumor safe reactions and influencing tumorigenesis.

In the event that influences antitumor insusceptibility fundamentally by expanding the self-restoration capacity of hematopoietic immature microorganisms and improving immunosuppression. Besides, the change of energy digestion brings about emotional down guideline of IGF-1 and up guideline of insulin-like development factor restricting protein-151 and expanded tumor cell autophagy and modified cell passing. These impacts are joined by a lessening in extracellular nucleoside triphosphate diphosphohydrolase articulation and ATP gathering, consequently hindering administrative T cells (Tregs) and invigorating cytotoxic T lymphocyte (CTL) capacities, which upgrades antitumor insusceptible reactions. Additionally, high articulation of heme oxygenase-1 (HO-1) in tumors can restrain tumor cell apoptosis and safe stimulatory impacts. Eminently, IF can diminish the statement of HO-1 in tumor cells and increment tumor cell apoptosis, just as upgrade incitement of CD8+ T cells by lessening the caloric inventory, which shapes a positive input circle of IF-prompted CD8+ T cell-cured slaughtering of tumor cells.

The impact of intermittent fasting (IF) on tumor insusceptible reactions. (A) Under ordinary conditions, the low autophagy level of tumor cells advances the declaration of CD73 and adenosine, which thusly influences the M2 polarization of tumor-related macrophages (TAMs). Also, the CD39 articulation and extracellular ATP increment, which invigorate Tregs and repress the elements of cytotoxic T lymphocytes (CTLs). Moreover, heme oxygenase 1 is exceptionally communicated in tumors and can hinder apoptosis and immune stimulatory impacts. The lactic corrosive delivered by tumor glycolysis hinders the capacity of normal executioner (NK) cells. (B) During IF, modified cell passing of tumor cells increments by means of autophagy and afterward decreases the declaration of CD73 and adenosine in the tumor microenvironment, which hinders the M2 polarization of TAMs. Besides, the outflow of CD39 in tumor cells and the amassing of extracellular ATP are restrained, in this manner repressing the capacity of administrative T cells and invigorating the capacity of CTLs. Additionally, IF can lessen the lactic corrosive level, in this manner reestablishing the capacity of NK cells. Initiation of the energy effectors AMPK and PPAR (a downstream atom of AMPK) restrain the creation of CCL2, accordingly decreasing the movement of monocytes from the bone marrow into the tumor microenvironment.

Moreover, IF can likewise manage antitumor resistant reactions by influencing the capacity and polarization of intrinsic invulnerable cells, like common executioner (NK) cells and tumor-related macrophages (TAMs). Lactic corrosive got from tumor cells can straightforwardly restrain NK cell-interceded executing and furthermore increment the quantity of myeloid-inferred silencer cells (MDSCs) to by implication repress NK cell capacities. In the event that can lessen the creation of lactic corrosive by tumor glycolysis, in this manner reestablishing the capacity of NK cells, diminishing the enhancement of MDSCs, and repressing tumor development. Moreover, the event of tumors is additionally firmly identified with polarization of neighborhood TAMs. Late examinations have shown that IF can diminish the digestion and fiery movement of monocytes because of the enactment of peroxisome proliferator-initiated receptor (PPAR) during fasting, and furthermore upgrade fix and safe reconnaissance in the body through actuation of AMPK. Moreover, intermittent fasting IF hinders the creation of chemokine C-C theme ligand 2 (CCL2) to diminish the quantity of aggravation related monocytes in the blood and tissues. In addition, IF can likewise inactivate the JAK1/STAT3 flagging pathway and decrease the declaration of CD73 and adenosine in the tumor microenvironment, which thusly influences the M2 polarization of TAMs and hinders tumor development.

The above investigations propose that IF can cause positive changes in the resistant cell populace, yet there are results that negate these examinations. For instance, IF in a lupus mouse model prompts the extension of Tregs. In addition, IF can compound intense resistance and conduct affliction because of incitement with the viral copy, poly. These discoveries propose that the impact of a particular IF routine on the turn of events and capacity of resistant cells is intricate and stays to be clarified.

Intermittent Fasting, Chemotherapy, and Radiotherapy

Past examinations have shown that fasting cycles joined with chemotherapy (CT) are reasonable and may moderate tumor movement and diminish CT-incited results in certain patients with various kinds of malignancy. The useful restorative impact of IF joined with CT on tumors show that IF upgrades the helpful impact of CT on tumors and furthermore essentially improves the irritation brought about by CT. Early examinations recommended that IF can create viable insusceptibility and decrease the frequency of disease and febrile neutropenia. Additionally, in creature models of foundational bacterial disease, intermittent fasting IF can repress irritation and secure psychological capacity. Further investigation has shown that IF can repress the declaration of proinflammatory cytokines, including RANTES/CCL5, TNF, IL 1, IL 6, and IL 10, and the incendiary body proteins NLRP1 and NLRP3 by enacting NF, in this way decreasing the frequency of irritation.

In any case, the specific instrument including the impacts of intermittent fasting IF joined with CT may likewise be unpredictable because of the fluctuated impact of IF on quality articulation. In the event that before CT has been appeared to shield the host from treatment poisonousness by decreasing the declaration of certain oncogenes, for example, RAS and the AKT flagging pathway. This decrease is intervened by diminishes in circling IGF-1 and glucose. Besides, IF-incited CR actuates different oncogenes in malignancy cells, initiates autophagy, and diminishes cell development rates while expanding the affectability of tumor cells to antimitotic drugs. Also, the impact of IF joined with CT on tumor development may rely totally upon the cell insusceptible framework, since CT joined with IF can't handle tumor development in nonthymic subject because of the absence of T lymphocytes.

Also, a few examinations have shown that IF expands malignancy sharpening to radiotherapy (RT) and broadens the endurance of starved trial creatures after various IF regimens. For instance, IF improves the endurance of subject with orthotropic pancreatic tumors exposed to deadly stomach radiation contrasted with controls with free access with food. Besides, IF doesn't influence radiation treatment intervened tumor cell slaughtering and upgrades H2AX staining after radiation treatment, recommending an extra gentle radio sharpening impact. Significantly, preclinical and some fundamental clinical information support the theory that IF could be used as an integral treatment to improve the result after RT, both as far as improved tumor control and a decreased likelihood of typical tissue complexities.

Albeit intermittent fasting IF joined with these customary anticancer treatments has shown promising outcomes in these essential investigations, more preclinical exploratory information are as yet required in light of the fact that clinical significance stays low because of inadequate human information, including not many clinical result contemplates, an absence of wellbeing information, and basically no randomized controlled preliminaries. Future investigations thusly need to zero in on wellbeing, and at last increment advantages to current treatments related with IF. Additionally, the capability of IF to upgrade the reaction to bring down dosages of CT and radiation treatment likewise ought to be additionally explored.

Intermittent Fasting and Immunotherapy of Tumor

By and by, there are no reports about intermittent fasting IF and tumor immunotherapy. In the tumor microenvironment, IF can diminish glucose take-up and glycolysis in tumor cells. Notwithstanding, effector T cells of antitumor safe reactions likewise depend on glycolysis to keep up their clonal development and capacity. Critically, considers have shown that insusceptible designated spot bar (ICB) treatment with PD-L1 antibodies specifically shields T cells from diminished glucose usage in the tumor microenvironment, which proposes that ICB joined with IF may turn into a promising clinical tumor treatment system. Nonetheless, IF can lessen the degree of coursing glucose and moderate the development of tumor cells. ICB is utilized to improve the energy digestion of T cells and keep up their function81 to accomplish an improved impact of clinical tumor immunotherapy. Notwithstanding, considering the intricacy of the energy digestion system set off by IF and the distinctions in ICB immunotherapy techniques, more forthcoming examinations are expected to portray the regimens and impacts of IF joined with tumor immunotherapy.

Intermittent Fasting and other therapies

One late examination showed that the mix of intermittent fasting IF and nutrient C was a promising intercession with low harmfulness, which could be tried in randomized clinical preliminaries against colorectal malignancy and potentially different tumors with KRAS changes. In particular, the anticancer movement of nutrient C is restricted by the up guideline of HO-1. Notwithstanding, IF selectivity turns around nutrient C-actuated up guideline of HO-1 and ferritin in KRAS-freak malignancy cells, thus expanding receptive iron, oxygen species, and cell passing, an impact that is additionally potentiated by CT. These discoveries demonstrate that IF joined with non-cytotoxic mixtures could be novel and promising medicines of tumors. Moreover, the connected movement on IF joined with tumor treatment was recorded.

2.5 Discussion

Momentum contemplates have shown that IF has a wide scope of impacts that improve energy digestion and the event of numerous infections; IF crucially affects tumor safe reactions, proposing that IF is arising as a promising technique in clinical tumor treatment. In any case, as a result of the intricacy of the impacts of IF on tissues and cell energy digestion, there are as yet numerous logical difficulties to be additionally tended to. In the current survey, we summed up three parts of these logical issues. (1) Regarding the system, what are the immediate impacts and components of IF on the turn of events and capacity of various tissue-explicit cells and resistant cells? For instance, one ongoing examination showed that 30-day IF was related with an anticancer serum proteomic signature, upregulated key administrative proteins related with glucose and lipid digestion, and influenced the circadian clock, DNA fix, cytoskeletal rebuilding, the invulnerable framework, and psychological capacity, and brought about a serum proteome that was defensive against malignant growth, metabolic disorder, and irritation. Moreover, it is significant that there are some unique healthful intercessions, which may prompt various impacts on physiological records including blood glucose, fatty oils, development chemical, insulin, and insulin-like development factor 1 (IGF-I). Distinctive clinical therapy techniques additionally may influence a definitive impacts of IF in malignant growth patients. Further examination is subsequently required before the utilization of IF as an intercession can be prescribed to build the personal satisfaction for tumor patients. (2) Regarding results, the various impacts of unmistakable IF regimens on the energy digestion of tumor patients remain generally obscure. To more readily screen the symptoms of IF, is it conceivable to normalize IF regimens for various malignancy medicines? One investigation announced that it will be important to test and normalize IF regimens by approaches that are like those performed for the endorsement of medications by the FDA, to permit these intercessions to be executed by a huge segment of the population.

(3) Regarding application, does IF intensify hunger or other unfriendly responses in tumor patients? A few examinations report that unhealthiness and sarcopenia habitually happen in malignant growth patients and negatively affect clinical results. The explanation might be driven by lacking food admission, diminished actual work, and catabolic metabolic confusions. The interaction in regards to the utilization of Intermittent fasting IF in disease patients ought to along these lines be more thorough, and assessment of major unfriendly clinical occasions (counting malnourishment, cachexia, conceivably a debilitated insusceptible framework, and expanded vulnerability to specific contaminations, which should be painstakingly observed) are an essential advance in deciding if healthful mediation is really advantageous. Also, in light of the fact that current examination has shown restricted wellbeing results, the discoveries are just valuable in growing longer-term preliminaries. Along these lines, future examinations should think about the danger of unhealthiness and sarcopenia, and the immunological and metabolic condition of the selected patients.

In synopsis, IF has arisen as a promising and useful asset in clinical tumor treatment. In any case, IF is a two sided deal that can influence tumorigenesis, increment safe reactions, and adjust the energy digestion of tumor patients. Moreover, there is an outstanding absence of examination on the impacts of IF joined with tumor immunotherapy and quality treatment. Accordingly, further exploration is required before the utilization of IF as a mediation can be prescribed to build the personal satisfaction for tumor patients. We accept that with additional clarification of the component of IF joined by the improvement of sub-atomic science, frameworks science, and super information, explicitly in regards to the connection among IF and tumor insusceptible reactions, IF will bring about new techniques for clinical tumor safe counteraction and treatment soon, with wide application possibilities.

Conclusion

Serum proteomic mark of 4-week intermittent fasting from day break to nightfall for over 14 hours daily added to the unthinking comprehension of the impact of intermittent fasting from sunrise to dusk on enemy of carcinogenesis, DNA fix, insulin flagging, humoral insusceptibility and expanded life span in subjects with metabolic condition. Our discoveries recommend that intermittent fasting from first light to dusk for four sequential weeks, which is in synchrony with circadian cadence and earth's revolution can be an assistant therapy in metabolic disorder and ought to be tried in the anticipation and therapy of metabolic condition actuated malignancies. Through and through, our discoveries are in accordance with the consequences of our previous investigation of 30-day sunrise to nightfall intermittent fasting led in sound subjects and establish the framework information for a randomized, controlled clinical preliminary of day break to dusk intermittent fasting in subjects with metabolic disorder.

Our investigation presents a novel dietary mediation technique and demonstrates that dragging out the length of the daily fasting stretch could be a straightforward and possible procedure to diminish bosom malignancy repeat. In this partner of patients with beginning phase bosom disease, a more extended daily fasting span was additionally connected with altogether lower centralizations of HbA1c and longer rest length. Given the relationship of daily fasting with glycemic control and rest, we conjecture that mediations to draw out the daily fasting span might actually diminish the danger of type 2 diabetes, cardiovascular infection, and different diseases. Consequently, discoveries from this investigation have wide and huge ramifications for general wellbeing. Randomized preliminaries are expected to enough test whether dragging out the daily fasting span can decrease the danger of ongoing sickness.

Lightning Source UK Ltd.
Milton Keynes UK
UKHW020630210521
384122UK00012B/723